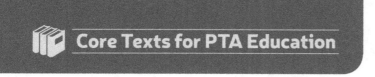

Core Texts for PTA Education

D1290382

Therapeutic Agents
for the **Physical Therapist Assistant**

SERIES EDITOR
MIA L. ERICKSON, PT, EDD, CHT, ATC

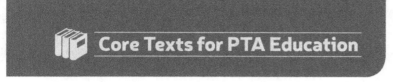

Core Texts for PTA Education

Therapeutic Agents
for the Physical Therapist Assistant

Jennifer Memolo, MA, PTA
The University of Alabama in Huntsville
Huntsville, Alabama

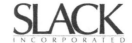

SLACK
INCORPORATED

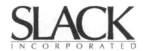

SLACK Incorporated
6900 Grove Road
Thorofare, NJ 08086 USA
856-848-1000   Fax: 856-848-6091
www.slackbooks.com
© 2022 by SLACK Incorporated

Senior Vice President: Stephanie Arasim Portnoy
Vice President, Editorial: Jennifer Kilpatrick
Vice President, Marketing: Mary Sasso
Acquisitions Editor: Tony Schiavo
Director of Editorial Operations: Jennifer Cahill
Vice President/Creative Director: Thomas Cavallaro
Cover Artist: Lori Shields
Project Editor: Dani Malady

Instructors: *Therapeutic Agents for the Physical Therapist Assistant* includes ancillary materials specifically available for faculty use. Included are *Instructor's Manual* and PowerPoint Slides. Please visit http://www.efacultylounge.com to obtain access.

Library of Congress Cataloging-in-Publication Data

Names: Memolo, Jennifer, author.
Title: Therapeutic agents for the physical therapist assistant / Jennifer Memolo.
Other titles: Core texts for PTA education
Description: Thorofare, NJ : SLACK Incorporated, [2022] | Series: Core texts for PTA education | Includes bibliographical references and index.
Identifiers: LCCN 2022006025 (print) | LCCN 2022006026 (ebook) | ISBN 9781630912420 (paperback) | ISBN 9781630912437 (epub) | ISBN 9781630912444
Subjects: MESH: Physical Therapy Modalities | Physical Therapist Assistants
Classification: LCC RM725 (print) | LCC RM725 (ebook) | NLM WB 460 | DDC 615.8/2--dc23/eng/20220211
LC record available at https://lccn.loc.gov/2022006025
LC ebook record available at https://lccn.loc.gov/2022006026

Printed in the United States of America.

Last digit is print number: 10 9 8 7 6 5 4 3 2 1

DEDICATION

To my mother, Wanda.

CONTENTS

Instructors: *Therapeutic Agents for the Physical Therapist Assistant* includes ancillary materials specifically available for faculty use. Included are *Instructor's Manual* and PowerPoint Slides. Please visit http://www.efacultylounge.com to obtain access.

ACKNOWLEDGMENTS

Many thanks to Clarkson College in Omaha, Nebraska, and the Physical Therapist Assistant program, to Shannon and Lane at the Physical Therapist Assistant program at Nebraska Methodist College in Omaha, and to Michelle at Lakeside Aquatic Physical Therapy in Omaha. Thanks also to my family for their patience and support, and to Tony and Mia for letting me write something new.

—*Jennifer Memolo, MA, PTA*

About the Author

Jennifer Memolo, MA, PTA lives in Huntsville, Alabama. She taught in the associate of science Physical Therapist Assistant program at Nebraska Methodist College in Omaha, Nebraska, and both the associate of science and bachelor of science Physical Therapist Assistant programs at Clarkson College in Omaha. She currently serves as the writer/editor for the Office of Development at The University of Alabama in Huntsville. She received her bachelor of arts degree in English at Birmingham-Southern College in Birmingham, Alabama, and then a master's in creative writing at East Carolina University in Greenville, North Carolina. She received her associate of science degree as a physical therapist assistant from Nash Community College, Rocky Mount, North Carolina, in 2008, at which time she moved to Omaha, where she worked and lived for 12 years. She has worked in inpatient rehabilitation, skilled nursing, and home health settings.

INTRODUCTION

Textbooks that address therapeutic agents (or modalities) can be challenging for physical therapist assistant students. Content in typical texts addresses issues more specific to physical therapists and what they need to know for evaluations and development of a plan of care. This text strives to focus on the needs of the physical therapist assistant, specifically the direct application of therapeutic agents. Each chapter will provide information about how the therapeutic agent works, indications and contradictions for use, the physiological effects of the agent on a person's body, and the parameters for setup and use. In addition, each chapter will contain review questions and documentation samples to facilitate improved patient care. This textbook is accompanied by an *Instructor's Manual* and PowerPoint presentations to assist with instruction and lab skill practice.

Unit I

Introduction

Chapter 1

An Introduction to Physical Agents

KEY TERMS Evidence-based research | Level of evidence | PICO(T) | Plan of care | Qualitative studies | Quantitative studies | Therapeutic agents

KEY ABBREVIATIONS APTA | PICO(T) | RCTs

CHAPTER OBJECTIVES

1. Explain the purpose of modalities in a patient's plan of care.
2. Describe and apply the components of evidence-based research to the application of modality interventions.
3. Create documentation supportive of intervention replication and reimbursement.

INTRODUCTION

The use of therapeutic agents (also referred to as *modalities* or *[bio]physical agents*) to influence a patient's performance during a physical therapy appointment is nothing new. Physical therapists and physical therapist assistants have been using heat, cold, electricity, and traction to improve a patient's pain or increase a patient's range of motion for decades. As such, it is important that a therapist understand how the agent works and what its effects are on the patient's body. One may find in their practice, for example, that some therapeutic agents are administered by therapy aides or technicians. However, owing to the importance of knowing how the modality works, why it is being used, why it should not be used, and what it is actually doing to the tissues, aides or techs are not appropriate to administer these interventions. Physical therapist assistants

are skilled clinicians with the knowledge and experience to carry out a physical therapist's plan of care, including the administration of therapeutic modalities.

AN OVERVIEW OF THERAPEUTIC AGENTS IN THE PLAN OF CARE

The Commission on Accreditation in Physical Therapy Education's *Standards and Required Elements for Accreditation of Physical Therapist Assistant Education Programs* stipulates in section 7D23 that physical therapist assistant programs should "demonstrate competence in implementing selected components of interventions identified in the plan of care established by the physical therapist," including biophysical agents.[1] These include "biofeedback, electrotherapeutic agents, compression therapies, cryotherapy, hydrotherapy, superficial and deep thermal agents, traction and light therapies."[1] In the American Physical Therapy Association's (APTA's) *Guide to Physical Therapist Practice*, these same therapeutic agents are listed as pertinent interventions for physical therapist assistants.[2] The *Guide* goes on to state that using these interventions can, among other things, assist muscle force generation and contraction, increase the rate of healing of open wounds and soft tissue, and modulate or decrease pain.[2] It is important to note that the APTA's Choosing Wisely campaign, which

Memolo J.
Therapeutic Agents for the Physical Therapist Assistant
(pp 3-7). © 2022 SLACK Incorporated.

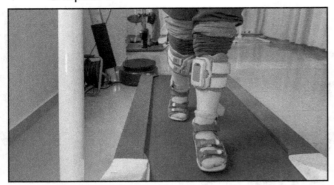

Figure 1-1. Use of modality to facilitate muscle contraction. (d13/Shutterstock.com)

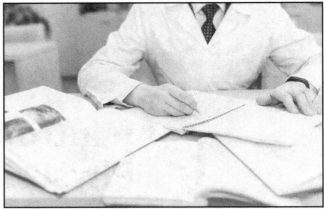

Figure 1-2. Use of research is key to effective interventions. (ARLOU_ANDREI/Shutterstock.com)

comprises 5 things therapists should avoid based on recent evidence, states that the use of (certain) therapeutic agents is not considered physical therapy when performed in the absence of other interventions unless there is documentation to support their exclusive use.[3] The use of a modality as the sole method of treatment is not considered physical therapy and is not beneficial. The patient may benefit from heat to increase range of motion in certain tissues, but the patient should then be stretched to fully profit from that modality. Patients may feel less pain after electrical stimulation, but then they should do their physical therapy exercises to gain strength. This is something to be driven home in any modalities class; the use of the therapeutic modality is most often a tool to help the patient do more. One may decrease the patient's pain before the therapy session so they will be able to do more activity, or one may end the session with something to decrease pain after a particularly strenuous session. One may use the modality to facilitate muscle activity, asking the patient to contract the muscle along with the machine (Figure 1-1). This is what differentiates a passive from an active treatment. A passive modality intervention is one that may relieve pain in the short term, but is not followed by or performed in combination with interventions that will potentially resolve the patient's pain (and mobility or function) in the long term. Active interventions, as described previously, use modalities to facilitate additional therapy interventions. Either way, a clinician should be able to document and provide rationale for any modality treatment provided.

Something else to consider is what to do when you see that your supervising physical therapist has included modalities in the plan of care. Medicare and other insurance companies are getting more and more specific in how they want documentation to look. In the past, it was not uncommon to see a physical therapist write "modalities as needed" in a plan of care. Now, a specific modality or a few options are more likely to be listed in the plan of care, such as "ultrasound to lower right back L3 to S1 for pain" or perhaps the more general "ultrasound and electrical stimulation for pain to lower right back." If there is a more general statement in the plan of care, this allows the

physical therapist assistant to select the best modality. A statement like "electrical stimulation for pain" narrows the options only a little, and again the physical therapist assistant can use their judgment to select the best option for the patient. Even if the plan of care is more specific, as in the aforementioned ultrasound examples, the physical therapist assistant is still able to make some choices on parameters when performing this intervention. The point is that, as a skilled clinician, the physical therapist assistant makes many specific choices about the modality interventions provided.

EVIDENCE-BASED RESEARCH

In any health care setting, the use of evidence to support interventions is important (Figure 1-2). With regard to therapeutic modalities, especially, the evidence that backs interventions can change based on the most current studies. One may find that different clinicians with varying backgrounds have equally differing thoughts on the correct parameters and indications for modality interventions. Even after a textbook is published, new studies may emerge that contradict or change the parameters listed in that textbook. This can be very frustrating to students who crave a concrete and unchanging list of modality parameters. However, it is important to know that the use of current studies to support or change the interventions is a key ingredient in maintaining the validity of modalities used in the clinic.

To this end, it is imperative that clinicians conduct their own research to determine whether an intervention is effective. This means the clinician should take into consideration both the patient and the diagnosis when researching a modality. For example, therapeutic ultrasound is considered an effective technique to promote wound healing according to some studies, whereas others are less certain. This could be due to the specific types of wounds being treated, such as chronic vs acute wounds or pressure ulcers vs surgical wounds. It could also be influenced by how the

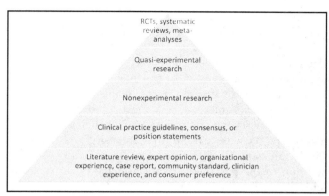

Figure 1-3. Levels of evidence.

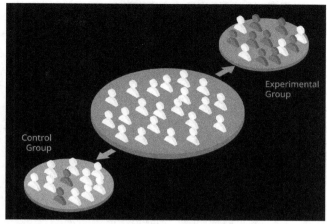

Figure 1-4. A randomized controlled trial. (Piscine26/Shutterstock.com)

studies are conducted.[4] More will be said about the types of studies shortly.

Additionally, some studies support the effectiveness of ultrasound for the treatment of some musculoskeletal soft-tissue pain (but not all diagnoses),[5] but its use for bone healing is contested.[6] Just because ultrasound may not be considered the best intervention for some diagnoses does not mean it is not effective in all situations.

As a part of conducting research to determine the best interventions, the clinician should know there are different levels of evidence. This means that not all research studies are equal, and one needs to think about the validity, reliability, and quality when looking at a study. Often these hierarchies of evidence are presented as a pyramid. Some have 5 levels of evidence, others 7. Regardless, one should be aware that some types of evidence are considered more reliable than others.

One such hierarchy is the Johns Hopkins hierarchy of evidence. Figure 1-3 depicts this hierarchy of evidence. At its top is level 1, which includes randomized controlled trials (RCTs), systematic reviews of RCTs, or meta-analyses of RCTs. RCTs require 3 criteria: random assignment of study participants into 2 or more groups, an intervention applied to at least 1 group, and a control group that does not receive treatment.[7] This is depicted in Figure 1-4. These studies are at the top of the pyramid because they have been deemed to have the highest level of reliability and validity, making the outcomes notable and worth considering for change. RCTs help to eliminate bias in a research study, and they also help to remove any confounding factors that might influence the study outcomes. Systematic reviews collate a large number of studies and then summarize and evaluate the studies' outcomes. This is often a way to make study results more accessible to readers, and because systematic reviews often collect outcomes from level 1 sources, the information is still considered reliable.

Level 2 in the hierarchy includes quasi-experimental studies or systematic reviews and meta-analyses of quasi-experimental studies. Quasi-experimental studies are those that include 1 or 2 of the criteria for an RCT.[7] Most often, quasi-experimental studies involve a control and experimental group, but a nonrandom method is used to assign each participant to each group.

Level 3 is composed of nonexperimental studies and their systematic reviews, systematic reviews of a combination of RCTs, quasi-experimental and nonexperimental studies, or nonexperimental studies only. Level 3 also includes qualitative studies or systematic reviews. Nonexperimental studies are those that cannot control the variables or participants and, therefore, rely more heavily on observation and interpretation. Qualitative studies are those that collect nonnumerical data, such as interviews or surveys. This is in contrast to quantitative studies, which collect numerical data so the researcher can describe or predict outcomes.

Level 4 includes expert opinion based on scientific or research evidence, clinical practice guideline, or consensus panels.[8] This level includes information from experts in the field, or those who have experience and knowledge of the topic based on their practice in the field. Level 5 includes the opinion of individual experts based on nonresearch evidence, including literature reviews, program evaluations, or case reports based on experiential and nonresearch evidence.[7] Literature reviews are a survey or summary of scholarly articles or books related to a specific question. Often, this question is referred to as a *PICO* or *PICO(T) question*, which stands for patient/problem, intervention, comparative intervention, outcome, and time. Sometimes, students are assigned to generate a PICO(T) question and then conduct a literature review to attempt to answer that question. For example, a therapy-related question might be: In teenage female patients who undergo a surgical anterior cruciate ligament repair (P), does the use of typical physical therapy exercises in combination with therapeutic ultrasound (I) vs the use of typical physical therapy exercises alone (C) yield improved mobility outcomes (O) when measured over a 4-week period (T)? One can fashion a PICO(T) question for almost any subject of interest, and a quick literature review might give insight on the best intervention for a diagnosis or patient population.

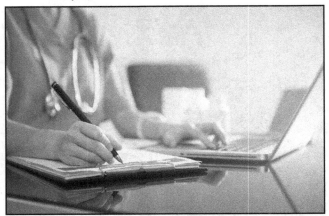

Figure 1-5. Documentation of modality interventions. (THICHA SATAPITANON/Shutterstock.com)

In addition to considering the hierarchy of evidence, a student, clinician, or researcher should look at the study's date; while some information from 10 years ago may still be accurate, it behooves the researcher to consult more recent sources. Some might suggest studies within the last 7 years are relevant; others recommend excluding studies more than 5 years old. This is due to the constant changes in health care technology and even the health care delivery system. The goal is to ensure that the research reviewed reflects the most current evidence and information.

A student or practicing clinician should be willing to research current evidence on therapy interventions and use that information to make the best choice regarding patient treatment. If a physical therapist assistant has found evidence that an intervention is deemed effective for a certain diagnosis, they can share the information with their supervising physical therapist, and together they can make the best choice for the diagnosis and the patient's needs.

In each chapter, this text will address what the current evidence says and provide students an opportunity to conduct research on the topic in the form of a PICO(T) question.

DOCUMENTATION

Subsequent chapters will have sample documentation to demonstrate how best to document and track patient performance and practice with respect to therapeutic modalities. This section provides a documentation checklist to follow when documenting a therapeutic modality. Including each of these items inspires confidence that the documentation is of high quality.

First, list the modality used. Here, one should be specific. Instead of writing "thermotherapy" or "electrical stimulation," state that a moist hot pack or interferential current was used on the patient. Next, indicate the patient position; was the patient prone, sidelying, or supine? Did they have pillows, towel rolls, or bolsters? Be specific.

Indicate the location of treatment. Again, be detailed in this account. Instead of writing "Left hip," indicate specifically where on the hip—use words like "superior" and "lateral" and refer to bony landmarks. One may even need to measure the distance of the treatment location to a bony landmark so the treatment is reproducible.

Treatment parameters are a must for documentation. Include every setting established. This includes duty cycle, megahertz, pulse rate, ramp time, intensity, and duration. The parameters will differ based on the modality used. In addition to the parameters, always include your purpose for treating the patient with a modality. Specify the goal to be accomplished. Something like "applied moist hot pack to lower lumbar spine L3-5 × 30 minutes with 8 layers to decrease pain and improve lumbar spine range of motion" is going to appeal to any insurance or Medicare reviewer.

Indicate the patient's response to the treatment as well as whether the treatment was effective. Did the patient report any subjective data as a result of the therapy? Did the patient say the hot pack was too hot (and were layers added), or did the patient show no signs of redness or blistering after the iontophoresis treatment? Report any changes (positive or negative) as it pertains to goals. If pain is the reason for treatment, get a pain scale report prior to treatment and again after; did the patient's pain decrease after using the transcutaneous electrical nerve stimulation unit? If needed, measure range of motion or strength. Include the goniometric measurements or manual muscle test results in the note.

Documenting the therapeutic modality intervention in detail will allow the therapist to be sure that Medicare or insurance will reimburse for the treatment, and it will allow the treatment session to be reproduced by either the same or a different therapist in the future. It is not always possible to remember what was done: If a physical therapist assistant sees 8 to 10 patients/day every day of the week, those treatment sessions blur together. If the therapist goes on vacation, they will want to know that their patients are receiving the treatment they need to get better. Proper documentation (Figure 1-5) will give the therapist that peace of mind. Table 1-1 lists all the components of an "O" section that should be included in the documentation.

CONCLUSION

This chapter only begins the discussion of why physical therapist assistants use therapeutic modalities to help their patients. Physical therapist assistants should be able to review a patient's plan of care and determine what modalities are appropriate and then apply those modalities to facilitate active therapeutic interventions. Part of being able to do that is keeping up to date on the most recent evidence regarding modality interventions and knowing what types of evidence best support those interventions. Physical therapist assistants should also be able to document those interventions in detail, including the rationale for each modality used and how those modalities play a role in the larger plan, to justify those interventions. The next chapters will discuss the specific modalities, some of which were briefly touched on in this chapter, as well as their indications, contraindications, and physiological effects.

Table 1-1
Documentation Components

Modality used—be specific
Patient position
Location of treatment—be specific
Treatment parameters
Purpose for treating
Patient response
Treatment effectiveness (progression toward goals)

REVIEW QUESTIONS

1. What are the primary modality interventions a physical therapist assistant should be familiar with?
2. What is the difference between active and passive modality interventions? Which intervention is more effective for patient care?
3. True/False: Physical therapist assistants can use their clinical judgment to choose modalities and/or parameters to treat a patient. Explain your answer.
4. What is the difference between level 1 and level 2 evidence sources?
5. Find two level 1 and two level 2 examples of evidence that either support (or do not support) the use of electrical stimulation to decrease pain.
6. You want to determine if using therapeutic ultrasound for the treatment of trigger points is the best choice for your patient. What would be an example of a level 1 evidence?
7. If documenting the effects of a therapeutic agent on edema, what is a measurement or objective assessment in documentation that will show whether the treatment is effective?
8. Create a delineated PICO(T) question based on the following information: use of low-level laser therapy to treat patients with stage III or worse pressure injuries. Once you have a PICO(T) question, conduct a brief database search for information; are there any current, high-level studies to address this question?

REFERENCES

1. Commission on Accreditation in Physical Therapy Education. Standards and required elements for accreditation of physical therapist assistant education programs. Published November 3, 2020. Accessed February 7, 2022. https://www.capteonline.org/globalassets/capte-docs/capte-pta-standards-required-elements.pdf
2. American Physical Therapist Association. *Guide to Physical Therapy Practice*. Published 2021. Accessed February 2, 2022. https://guide.apta.org/interventions/categories-interventions/biophysical-agents
3. American Physical Therapist Association. *Choosing Wisely*. Published September 15, 2014. Accessed January 11, 2020. www.choosingwisely.org
4. Kotronis G, Vas PRJ. Ultrasound devices to treat chronic wounds: the current level of evidence. *Int J Low Extrem Wounds*. 2020;19(4):341-349.
5. Papadopoulos ES, Mani R. The role of ultrasound therapy in the management of musculoskeletal soft tissue pain. *Int J Low Extrem Wounds*. 2020;19(4):350-358.
6. Buarque de Gusmão CV, Batista NA, Vidotta Lemes VT, et al. Effect of low-intensity pulsed ultrasound stimulation, extracorporeal shockwaves and radial pressure waves on Akt, BMP-2, ERK-2, FAK and TGF-β1 during bone healing in rat tibial defects. *Ultrasound Med Biol*. 2019;45(8):2140-2161.
7. Glasofer A, Townsend AB. Determining the level of evidence: experimental research appraisal. *Nurs Crit Care (Ambler)*. 2019;14(6):22-25.
8. Johns Hopkins University. Johns Hopkins nursing evidence-based practice. Appendix C: evidence level and quality guide. 2017. Accessed May 20, 2021. www.hopkinsmedicine.org/evidence-based-practice/_docs/appendix_c_evidence_level_quality_guide.pdf

Chapter 2

Modality Categories and Indications

KEY TERMS Acute pain | Chronic pain | Clonus | Conversion | Cryotherapy | Deep somatic pain | Electrical stimulation | Electromagnetic agents | Endorphins | Flaccidity | Gate Control theory | Hydrotherapy | Hypertonic | Hypotonic | Mechanical agents | Nociceptors | Radiating pain | Radiation | Referred pain | Rigidity | Sclerotome | Spasticity | Thermal agents | Thermotherapy

KEY ABBREVIATIONS ADL | CDC | CHF | CVA | EMG | FES | IFC | NIDA | NMES | PAG | PENS | ROM | SG | TBI | TENS

CHAPTER OBJECTIVES

1. Describe the categories and types of therapeutic agents.
2. Discuss how the various agents transfer energy to the tissues.
3. Explain the 4 primary indications for using therapeutic agents.

INTRODUCTION

When working in the field, therapists need to be able to identify the best intervention for the patient. As discussed in the previous chapter, this decision relies heavily on staying current on the most recent research about when and how to use a modality. Another important aspect is knowing what category each modality falls under and how that modality transfers energy to the tissues to yield the desired outcome. Physical therapist assistants must know the primary indications for modalities in order to make the best decision for their patients' care.

THERAPEUTIC AGENT CATEGORIES AND TYPES

For the purposes of this book, therapeutic agents have been categorized by the type of energy they deliver. There are other ways to categorize modalities; one may consider how the energy is transferred, and one might also consider the depth of penetration for each modality (Tables 2-1 and 2-2). These specifics will be addressed, but first this chapter will discuss what type of energy each modality delivers and some of the specific examples of each (Table 2-3).

Thermal agents include thermotherapy and cryotherapy, such as shown in Figure 2-1. Thermotherapy provides superficial heat to the tissues and includes superficial moist heat, paraffin, and fluidotherapy. Warm whirlpool can be included in this section as it does technically provide superficial heating to the body, but in this text, it will be covered in more detail in the Hydrotherapy chapter (Chapter 6). Cryotherapy provides superficial cooling to the tissues, and includes interventions such as ice pack, gel pack, ice massage, cryocuff, ice immersion, and contrast bath. A cold whirlpool can be classified as cryotherapy, but it will also be addressed in Chapter 6.

Memolo J.
Therapeutic Agents for the Physical Therapist Assistant
(pp 9-18). © 2022 SLACK Incorporated.

Table 2-1
Modality Methods of Energy Transfer

How Energy Is Transferred	Examples of Modalities
Conduction	Moist hot pack, paraffin, ice pack, cold pack, ice massage, cryocuff, contrast bath, ice immersion
Convection	Fluidotherapy, warm/cold whirlpool
Conversion	Ultrasound/phonophoresis, diathermy
Evaporation	Vapocoolant spray
Radiation	UV, infrared, laser
Electricity	NMES, TENS, IFC, EMG biofeedback
Mechanical	Soft-tissue mobilization, traction, compression, hydrotherapy

Table 2-2
Table for Depth of Penetration

Modality	Depth of Penetration
Moist hot pack, paraffin ice pack, cold pack, ice massage, cryocuff, contrast bath, vapo-coolant spray, ice immersion	1 to 2 cm
Ultrasound (continuous); diathermy (continuous)	5 cm
Infrared	1.5 inches (3.8 cm)
Low-level laser therapy	5 cm

Table 2-3
Therapeutic Agents Categorized by Energy

Thermal Energy	• Superficial heat • Cryotherapy
Sound Energy	• Ultrasound • Phonophoresis
Mechanical	• Hydrotherapy • Traction • Compression • Manual therapy
Electrical and Electromagnetic Therapy	• Electrotherapy • Shortwave diathermy • LASER, infrared, and ultraviolet therapies

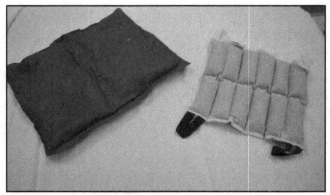

Figure 2-1. Example of a moist hot pack and cold pack.

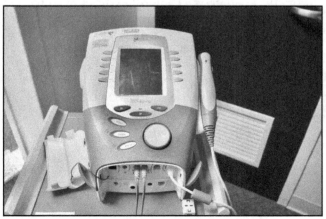

Figure 2-2. Ultrasound machine.

Figure 2-2 shows sound agents such as ultrasound and phonophoresis. Sound energy modalities use acoustic waves to generate energy and are sound waves that cannot be heard by the human ear. Ultrasound can create heat to decrease pain or improve tissue extensibility, but it can also promote healing of tissues. Phonophoresis is a form

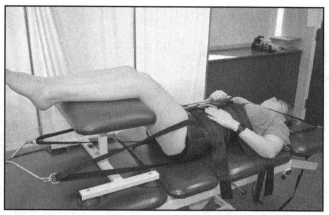

Figure 2-4. Patient on a traction table.

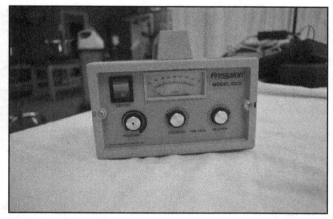

Figure 2-5. Compression unit.

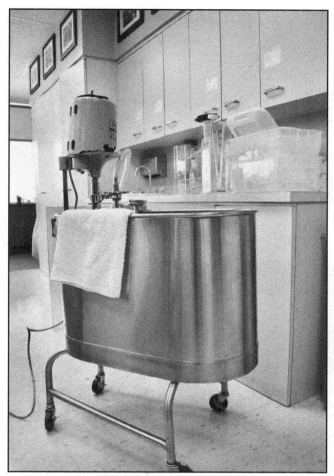

Figure 2-3. Hydrotherapy tub.

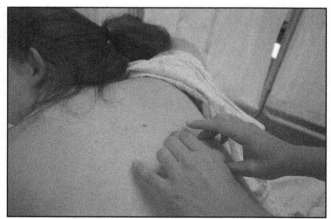

Figure 2-6. Massage.

of ultrasound that uses acoustic waves to allow medicine to efficiently penetrate the tissues, possibly eliminating the need for a systemic oral medication or injection.

Mechanical agents include hydrotherapy, traction, compression, and soft-tissue mobilization. All of these modalities involve some kind of force applied to the tissues for a therapeutic effect. Hydrotherapy includes warm or cold whirlpools, but it also includes using water for wound care interventions and either body-part or whole-body immersion to decrease pain or improve joint or tissue extensibility. Figure 2-3 shows a hydrotherapy whirlpool tub. Traction can be either manual or mechanical, and it involves pulling apart (distracting) joints to create space for the purposes of minimizing nerve compression or muscle tightness. Figure 2-4 shows a traction set-up. Compression (Figure 2-5) includes the use of wraps and garments or machines to push excess fluid in an area toward the heart; this could be used for anything from a sprained ankle to blood clot prevention to lymphedema treatment. Soft-tissue mobilization includes general massage techniques (Figure 2-6) as well as specialized interventions such as myofascial release and some joint mobilizations.

Electrical agents include interventions to help decrease pain, such as transcutaneous electrical nerve stimulation (TENS) and interferential current therapy (IFC), and stimulation to make muscles contract, such as neuromuscular electrical stimulation (NMES) or patterned electrical neuromuscular stimulation (PENS). Figure 2-7 shows an example of an electrical stimulation unit. Electrical stimulation

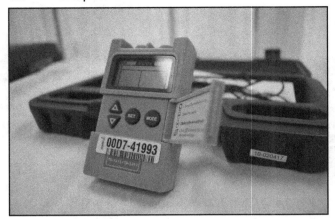

Figure 2-7. Electrical stimulation unit.

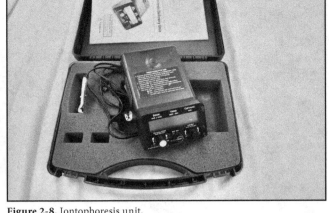

Figure 2-8. Iontophoresis unit.

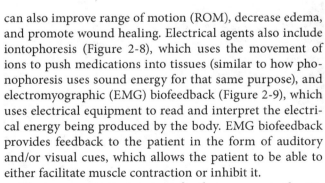

Figure 2-9. Biofeedback unit.

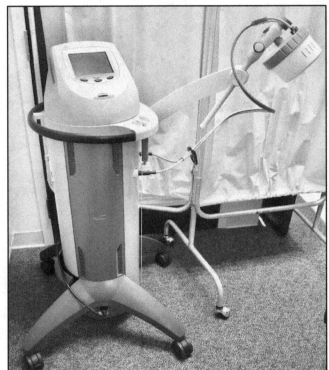

Figure 2-10. Diathermy machine.

can also improve range of motion (ROM), decrease edema, and promote wound healing. Electrical agents also include iontophoresis (Figure 2-8), which uses the movement of ions to push medications into tissues (similar to how phonophoresis uses sound energy for that same purpose), and electromyographic (EMG) biofeedback (Figure 2-9), which uses electrical equipment to read and interpret the electrical energy being produced by the body. EMG biofeedback provides feedback to the patient in the form of auditory and/or visual cues, which allows the patient to be able to either facilitate muscle contraction or inhibit it.

Electromagnetic agents transfer their energy to the tissues via radiation. Shortwave diathermy, lasers, infrared light, and ultraviolet (UV) light fall under this category. Like ultrasound, shortwave diathermy (Figure 2-10) can either deliver heat or can promote tissue healing. LASER, which is an acronym for "light amplification by stimulated emission of radiation," is classified as a cold laser and is used for healing and pain management. Figure 2-11 shows a laser unit. Infrared is considered a thermal modality, but it uses radiation to transmit energy. It is often used in the treatment of neuropathy or to heat tissues via a lamp. UV light is also delivered via a light source; care must be taken

to prevent burning the patient. The most common use of UV light in physical therapy is in the treatment of wounds.

Basic Indications for Therapeutic Agents

As mentioned previously, the *Guide to Physical Therapist Practice* lists the various indications for using therapeutic agents with patients. Reasons listed include "to assist muscle force generation and contraction; decrease unwanted muscular activity; increase the rate of healing of open

Table 2-4	
Therapeutic Modality Indications	
Therapeutic Modality	Indications
Electrical stimulation—high volt	Wounds, edema
Electrical stimulation—direct current	Pain, inflammation, swelling, wounds
Electrical stimulation—interferential	Pain
Electrical stimulation—Russian	Muscle strengthening, ROM
Shortwave diathermy	Pain, acute or chronic soft-tissue injuries
Cryotherapy	Pain, swelling (acute or chronic)
Thermotherapy	Pain, chronic injuries, healing, ROM
Ultrasound/phonophoresis	Pain, wound healing, bone healing
Laser	Pain, wound healing
Hydrotherapy	Wound healing, pain, used for exercise
Traction	Joint/vertebral pain, headaches
Soft-tissue mobilization/manual techniques	Pain, swelling, limited ROM
Compression	Swelling/edema, limited ROM
UV light	Wound healing, skin conditions
Infrared light	Pain, chronic injuries

wounds and soft tissue; maintain strength after injury or surgery; modulate or decrease pain; reduce or eliminate edema; improve circulation; decrease inflammation, connective tissue extensibility, or restriction associated with musculoskeletal injury or circulatory dysfunction; increase joint mobility, muscle performance, and neuromuscular performance; increase tissue perfusion and remodel scar tissue; and treat skin conditions."[1]

These indications can be combined into 5 primary categories that we will discuss in more detail here. They include alteration of pain, decreasing inflammation, promoting wound healing, modifying muscle tone, and altering tissue extensibility. Table 2-4 details the indications for all therapeutic agents covered in this text.

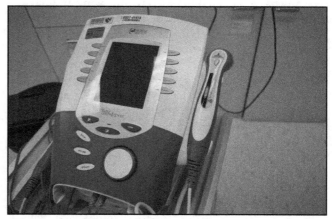

Figure 2-11. Laser unit.

Alteration of Pain Threshold

Pain is one of the primary reasons people come to physical therapy. A patient may have plantar fasciitis and it hurts to walk, while another pulled a muscle in their back getting groceries. A patient may have had knee surgery and it hurts to move it. Pain is also a very complex sensation, culminating from a combination of sensory and psychological input, and it is a sensation that originates from the evolutionary need to stay alive. Pain tells us something is wrong and helps us avoid doing something that may cost us our mobility or livelihood.

Pain is also the primary reason patients take over-the-counter or prescription medications. While prescription pain medications can sometimes be necessary to function, health care providers are trying to move away from prescribing pain medications as a long-term solution to pain. According to the National Institute on Drug Abuse (NIDA), more than 130 people/day die in the United States after overdosing on opioids.[2] Drugs like heroin and fentanyl are included in that statistic, but prescription pain relievers are a major part of the problem. The NIDA website clarifies that, starting in the late 1990s, more prescription pain medications were being prescribed with no education about the possibility of addiction.[2] The result was that the number of people addicted to opioids increased and so, too, did the rate of overdoses. We are now in what is referred to as an *opioid crisis*, and the NIDA is working with the United States Department of Health and Human Services (HHS) to change this. Two of the priorities of the NIDA and HHS are to provide "support for cutting-edge research on pain and addiction" and to advance "better practices for pain management."[2] The Centers for Disease Control and Prevention (CDC) echoes this sentiment in its "CDC Guideline for Prescribing Opioids for Chronic Pain" factsheet, which states that, before starting opioids to treat chronic pain, patients should "consider ways to manage pain that do not include opioids, such as physical therapy."[3] The American Physical Therapy Association wrote a white paper, which is an informational document used to promote or highlight the features of a solution or service, on how physical therapy providers can help manage pain through the use of regular exercise, manual therapy, stress management, sleep hygiene, and pain neuroscience education.[4]

Therapeutic agents can help modulate pain in a variety of ways. First, one must understand the types of pain and the basics of how pain signals are transmitted from the body to the brain.

Types of Pain

Pain can be divided into several different categories. One primary differentiation is acute vs chronic pain. Acute pain typically has a sudden onset directly following an injury or tissue damage. Think about the pain associated immediately after spraining your ankle or cutting your finger with a knife. Chronic pain lasts more than 6 months; this may be the pain associated with a knee injury that has not healed well or the pain accompanying a cancer diagnosis.

Neuropathic pain is typically caused by damage to the somatosensory system and is accompanied by tissue injury.[5] The peripheral nerve fibers themselves are damaged as a result of the injury, causing them to send inaccurate signals to the brain. This results in altered function at the site of the injury as well in surrounding areas.[5]

Another type of pain is referred pain. Referred pain can be acute or chronic, and its identifying factor is that the pain felt is distant from the actual source of the pain. Think about the classic signs and symptoms for a heart attack: chest pain, jaw pain, arm pain, nausea. With exception of the chest pain, these painful symptoms are not directly near the heart. Radiating pain, in contrast, is pain that travels down the pathway of a nerve. For example, injury or compression of the sciatic nerve presents as pain that travels from the buttocks down the back of the leg and into the foot on the affected side. Radiating pain can also be acute or chronic.

A final type of pain worth noting is deep somatic pain. This pain is affiliated with a sclerotome, or a segment of bone innervated by a spinal segment. It can fall under the acute or chronic definition.

How Pain Is Perceived

There is a saying: "You don't see with your eyes, you see with your brain." That is, the nerves in one's eyes send information to the brain, and the brain interprets that information into visual information. The same thing applies to pain. The nerves in one's body pick up pain sensations and send them to the brain, where they are then interpreted as pain. There are nociceptors, or peripheral pain receptors, that pick up pain sensations and transmit that information to the brain. These can be subdivided generally into $A\delta$ (delta) and C fibers. Although $A\delta$ and C fibers are both considered slower conducting, $A\delta$ fibers are the faster of the 2 (because of myelination) and transmit information related to pain, temperature, and some mechanical changes. Pain received through $A\delta$ fibers is sharp, localized, and brief (such as the pain of a pinprick). Sensations received through C fibers, the slower (and unmyelinated) of the 2, include pain, temperature, and itch, and it is dull, aching, or throbbing, and it is poorly localized. If either of these nerve fibers is stimulated, the corresponding pain signal is sent to the brain.

How does that work? According to Melzack and Wall,[6] the gate in the spinal cord is the substantia gelatinosa (SG); it modulates the transmission of sensory information from the afferent (sensory) neurons to the transmission (T) cells. Small fiber activity (that of the $A\delta$ and C fibers) opens the gate and leads to pain signals being transmitted to the primary sensory cortex in the brain. Large fiber activity inhibits or closes the gate; examples include fibers that sense muscle length, touch, and vibration.

So let's put this in action. First, let's say someone bangs their shin on the coffee table. The nociceptors in the tissue pick up that sensation. In this situation, the $A\delta$ fibers are likely to be triggered first, but the dull ache felt afterward is attributed to C fibers. The pain sensation travels up from the periphery to the dorsal horn of the spinal cord. Inside this area of the spinal cord is the gating mechanism that either allows pain signals to get to the brain or inhibits that stimuli. The T cells are either excited by the pain fibers or repressed by inhibitory neurons in the SG of the spinal cord. When the nociceptors are stimulated by the force of the table, the inhibitory neurons in the SG are inactivated (while the T cells are excited) and the signal of pain is sent up the cord to the primary sensory cortex of the brain via a neurotransmitter called *substance P*. Thus—ouch!

Gate Control Theory

Now that pain perception has been explained, the various theories related to how physical therapy can modulate pain via therapeutic agents can be discussed. The first theory is the Gate Control theory. Proposed by Melzack and Wall in 1965,[6] the Gate Control theory suggests that because there is a gating system in the SG, that gate can be opened or closed based on superficial sensory information.[5]

In addition to Aδ and C fibers, there are also Aβ fibers. These are sensory fibers that transmit touch and vibration. These fibers are large and myelinated, and sensory information travels faster than on the Aδ and C fibers. Thus, when the Aβ fibers are stimulated, the signal travels rapidly along the (relatively large and myelinated) fibers to the SG in the dorsal horn of the spinal cord. There, they inhibit the Aδ and C fibers and close the gate; no substance P is released and the only sensation sent up to the primary sensory cortex is the touch or vibration sensation of the Aβ fibers.

Now go back to banging the shin. It hurts! So what does one do? Likely one rubs the shin, and this makes it feel (a little) better. Why? The Aβ fibers are being activated. The sensation of touch travels to the SG in the spinal cord, closes the gate, and allows only the touch sensation to make it to the brain. Therapeutic interventions such as moist hot packs or IFC use the Gate Control theory to mask or block the pain signals.

Descending Pain Control Theory

According to Stamford,[7] pain sensations are not only an ascending transmission, but they are also controlled by the higher centers of the brain. These pathways originate in the thalamus and brainstem and the periaqueductal gray matter in the midbrain and are activated by adverse emotions, such as fear or stress, as well as previous experiences. For example, if one had a bad or painful experience at the dentist at a previous appointment, one would likely feel anxiety about the next appointment. Heightened anxiety and stress can, in turn, heighten the sense of pain. Serotonin, noradrenaline, and endogenous opiates are the main neurotransmitters in this theory.[7] These neurotransmitters, particularly serotonin, suppress the release of substance P, thus blocking the pain signal. This makes sense because each of these neurotransmitters works to regulate anxiety, allow the body to perform well in stressful conditions, or increase a sense of well-being.

Opiate (Endogenous Opioid) Theory

The body makes its own opiates, called *endorphins*. These are released by the pituitary gland and hypothalamus in response to strenuous exercise, excitement, pain, and orgasm.[8] It is like going for a long run: painful at first, but then one gets that "runner's high" that helps push through and keep on running. This is also why exercise can improve a person's mood. When the body encounters stress or pain, endorphins are released to provide an analgesic effect.[8] This same analgesic effect can be stimulated by certain therapeutic agents that cause a noxious stimulus; acupuncture TENS, for example, causes a pricking sensation, and the premise is that the noxious stimulus causes the body to create its own endorphins to decrease the pain.

Decreased Inflammation

This section will review the phases of healing. Healing can be divided into the inflammation phase, proliferation phase, and the remodeling or maturation phase.[9] During the inflammation phase, which generally lasts the first 24 to 48 hours, the blood vessels initially vasoconstrict to control blood loss until a scab or clot has formed. Then the vessels dilate to allow cells necessary for healing to reach the area of injury.[7] Here, we see the cardinal signs of inflammation: swelling, redness, warmth, and pain.

During the proliferation phase, which can last up to 24 days after the injury, fibroblasts are generating new tissue and a new blood supply is being generated.[9] Finally, the remodeling or maturation phase involves the wound shrinking as the edges contract while scar tissue is laid down and reorganized to be smaller and stronger. This can last up to 2 to 3 years after the injury.[9]

There are various things that can affect or impede healing, and these should be taken into consideration when contemplating the use of therapeutic agents to promote healing. These include the extent of the injury; the amount of swelling; the amount of bleeding; the blood supply available; the medications used by the patient; the patient's health, age, and nutritional status; the risk for or presence of infection; the risk for excessive scarring (such as keloids or hypertrophic scars); and the wound edges (ie, are they even and able to be approximated, or jagged and separated).

Promote Wound Healing

Wounds can be healed by a variety of means. If the wound edges are easily approximated and clean, sutures, staples, glue, or even butterfly closures will likely do the trick. This is called *healing by first intention*. However, some wounds are not so easily handled; the patient may have complicating factors as listed previously that will require more than stitches to repair the injury. In this case, the use of therapeutic agents is an option.

Modification of Muscle Tone

Muscle Tone

Muscle tone can be generally subdivided into hypertonic or hypotonic. Both conditions can lead to decreased function and pain. A muscle with too much tone may prevent full ROM and will limit mobility and function; too little tone can lead to pain, subluxations, and again, a lack of function. The increase or lack of muscle tone is involuntary. It may be the result of a neurological injury, such as a cerebral vascular accident, a traumatic brain injury, or Parkinson disease. The patient may also have increased or decreased tone due to a soft-tissue injury or prolonged positioning/postures.

Hypertonic muscle tone means that the muscle has too much tone, or that the muscle (and corresponding joints) are difficult to move. Hypertonicity includes descriptor

Table 2-5
Negative Side Effects of Hypertonicity
Pain
Contractures
Abnormal posturing
Increased work for caregivers
Development of altered movement patterns
Skin breakdown/wounds
Decreased activities of daily living, mobility

Table 2-6
Negative Side Effects of Hypotonicity
Poor posture
Decreased ability to move
Increased work for caregivers
Decreased activities of daily living, mobility
Pain
Skin breakdown/wounds
Decreased cardiopulmonary endurance
Compromised joint integrity

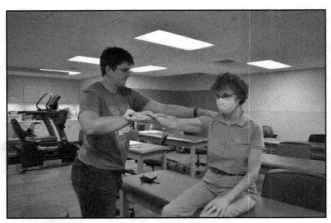

Figure 2-12. Manual muscle testing simulation.

words such as rigidity, spasticity, and clonus. Rigidity is when muscles are resistant to stretch regardless of the speed of movement, while spasticity is when the resistance to stretch is velocity dependent. Clonus is when the patient demonstrates rhythmic beats of muscle contractions in response to a quick stretch. Each of these impairs movement and functional activities and comes with a host of repercussions. Potentially negative effects of hypertonicity are listed in Table 2-5.

Hypotonicity, in contrast, means that the muscle is slack or flaccid. Hypotonic muscles are usually described as having a lack of tone or absence of resistance to stretch. Paresis is a type of muscle weakness, typically due to an injury. Paralysis is another word affiliated with hypotonicity, but is the complete loss of voluntary muscle contraction. There are some consequences of hypotonicity that are unique, but many overlap with hypertonicity, and they all contribute to a decrease in function and quality of life. Table 2-6 lists the negative effects of hypotonicity.

Just as with pain and wounds or tissue healing, therapeutic agents can be used to increase or decrease abnormal muscle tone. The use of heat (moist heat, paraffin, continuous ultrasound, continuous shortwave diathermy, warm whirlpool) can help relax a hypertonic muscle. Quick icing or a cold whirlpool may facilitate tone in a

hypotonic muscle. Electrical stimulation can be used to fatigue a hypertonic muscle (the agonist) or to stimulate a muscle to increase tone.[10] Massage may be relaxing to tonic musculature, and certain forms of traction may also alleviate tonic positioning. EMG biofeedback can provide information to the patient on what is happening in the muscle to facilitate either contraction or relaxation, depending on the need.

Muscle Strengthening

Just as various therapeutic modalities can influence the tone of a muscle, so can they affect muscle strength. It is very common to see certain therapeutic agents used in the clinic to improve or increase muscle strength. Most commonly, some form of electrical stimulation is used to facilitate muscle movement and improve strength. Examples include NMES, functional electrical stimulation (FES), or PENS. Electrical stimulation activates the fast twitch fibers in a muscle to facilitate a muscular contraction; very often, the patient is instructed to participate with the electrical stimulation machine to contract the muscle when the unit contracts the muscle. As in the case with FES, the electrical stimulation is used while performing a functional task, such as reaching for items or gait training.[11] Therapists can perform manual muscle testing (Figure 2-12) as well as other assessments to determine how much the muscle strength is improving.

Another therapeutic agent used to improve muscle strength is EMG biofeedback. While EMG biofeedback does not directly stimulate the muscles, it does read what electrical activity is being generated by the muscles and provides that feedback to the patient. Patients can then see what muscle activity they are doing and make adjustments or changes to improve the muscle contraction.

Alteration of Tissue Extensibility

Maintaining normal ROM for joints is important for the patient to perform activities of daily living. As a clinician, one needs to be able to measure the patient's ROM and know what is normal and what is not. Aside from a few exceptions, such as patients with spinal cord injuries, every joint should have as close to normal ROM as possible for full function. However, tissue restrictions are common in patients for a variety of reasons. The patient may have had a surgery and scar tissue or pain is limiting ROM. Pain or the fear of pain can lead to muscle guarding or disuse, affecting full ROM in a joint. Perhaps the patient has poor posture, causing tightness in some areas and leading to limited ROM in specific joints. Soft-tissue injuries such as sprains and strains can limit ROM because of pain and edema. Edema caused by lymphedema or other illnesses could restrict ROM as well.

A patient may have capsular restriction in a joint, leading to impaired movement in multiple planes. These restrictions can be caused by joint effusion, fibrosis, or inflammation related to arthritis or acute injury. A joint may also have restrictions related to adhesions or extra-articular lesions in a portion of the joint, limiting some but not all planes of movement. The patient may have injury or dysfunction of the muscle, the musculotendinous junction, or the tendon connected to that muscle, in which case the patient will demonstrate an ROM restriction during active ROM, whereas injury to skin, fascia, ligaments, bursa, cartilage, bone, or nerves results in limited passive ROM.

ROM can also be affected by pathological conditions, such as contractures, adhesions, bony changes in the joint, herniations, or even muscle weakness (possibly due to a neurological event).

ROM can be assessed in a variety of ways, although the most common is with a goniometer. Figure 2-13 shows a goniometric measurement being taken. Once ROM has been identified as limited in a certain joint, one must consider the causes.

Therapeutic agents can help mitigate the loss of ROM due to these various causes. NMES can increase ROM by facilitating muscle contractions. Thermal agents such as moist heat, continuous ultrasound, continuous shortwave diathermy, or warm whirlpool can decrease joint fluid viscosity and improve muscle elasticity to promote improved ROM. Thermotherapy, cryotherapy, and electrical stimulation such as TENS or IFC can decrease pain related to stretching, allowing for improved ROM. Depending on the cause of the limitation, therapeutic agents can assist in increasing limited ROM.

Edema

ROM can be limited for many reasons, as listed previously; edema or effusion can be set aside as a separate cause for limited tissue extensibility. Edema is generally described as the swelling that occurs outside a joint, while effusion is the swelling that occurs within a joint. Edema can be caused by a variety of pathologies; a patient could sprain their ankle and have acute swelling at the site of injury, or one could have congestive heart failure and increased swelling due to

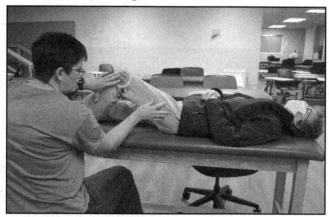
Figure 2-13. Goniometric measurement simulation.

the difficulty of the heart to pump fluids. Keeping in mind the contraindications, various forms of compression can control or even reverse edema. Compression can be static in the form of wrapping or garments, or it can be performed via intermittent compression machines. Cryotherapy is often used to address the swelling associated with acute injuries such as sprains and strains.

CONCLUSION

When a therapist understands the basic categories of modalities, as well as how those modalities work, that therapist can make the best choice of how to treat their patient. While there are more than 4 indications for any given modality, one will find that many patients' diagnoses fall under one of the primary indications discussed in this chapter. The subsequent chapters of this text will look at each modality in detail.

There are some other aspects of modality application one must know before administering these interventions. The physical therapist assistant should know the indications and contraindications for each specific modality. For example, a wound in the inflammatory phase might respond best to ice or other cryotherapy interventions; heat is generally contraindicated in acute conditions, as you will read about in another chapter.[9] Once the wound is considered subacute (not in the acute inflammatory phase), heating may be appropriate. Prolonged use of ice may even impede the important and necessary aspects of inflammation that lead to healing and a reduction in infection.[9] Knowing these indications and contraindications allows the clinician to provide the best intervention when the patient needs it.

Once contraindications have been cleared and the wound's phase of healing has been determined, one can consider what each modality might do for a wound depending on the needs. See Table 2-7 for a clinical justification chart on selecting the correct modality for wound care.

Table 2-7
Clinical Justification for Wound Care

Is the Wound Infected?	• Electrical stimulation • UV light
Is the Wound Due to Venous Insufficiency?	• Intermittent compression
Is the Wound in the Inflammatory Phase?	• Cryotherapy • Ultrasound (pulsed) • Laser
Does the Wound Require Debridement/Cleansing?	• Hydrotherapy
Is the Wound Due to Arterial Insufficiency?	• Electrical stimulation

Modalities that are most commonly used for wound care include electrical stimulation, ultrasound, UV light, hydrotherapy, shortwave diathermy, and laser. The specifics of each of these will be addressed in their corresponding chapters.

REVIEW QUESTIONS

1. What are the types of energy produced by therapeutic agents?
2. List 3 reasons one might use a therapeutic agent to treat a patient per the physical therapist's plan of care.
3. What are the 4 primary indications for using therapeutic agents?
4. Which therapeutic agent uses acoustic energy?
5. What are the phases of healing when a tissue is injured?
6. When healing tissue in the inflammatory phase of healing, what therapeutic agents are appropriate?
7. What modalities would be appropriate to improve tissue extensibility?
8. Name the modalities that could address acute pain. What about chronic pain?

REFERENCES

1. American Physical Therapy Association. *Guide to Physical Therapist Practice 3.0.* Published August 1, 2014. Accessed June 20, 2019. http://guidetoptpractice.apta.org/content/1/SEC35.body
2. National Institute on Drug Abuse. *Opioid Overdose Crisis.* Published January 2019. Accessed June 20, 2019. https://www.drugabuse.gov/drugs-abuse/opioids/opioid-overdose-crisis
3. Centers for Disease Control and Prevention. CDC guideline for prescribing opioids for chronic pain. Published April 17, 2019. Accessed June 20, 2019. https://www.cdc.gov/drugoverdose/pdf/guidelines_at-a-glance-a.pdf
4. American Physical Therapy Association. Beyond opioids: how physical therapy can transform pain management to improve health. Published 2018. Accessed June 20, 2019. http://www.apta.org/uploadedFiles/APTAorg/Advocacy/Federal/Legislative_Issues/Opioid/APTAOpioidWhitePaper.pdf
5. American Chronic Pain Association. Neuropathic pain. Published 2019. Accessed January 11, 2020. www.theacpa.org
6. Melzack R, Wall PD. Pain mechanisms: a new theory. *Science.* 1965;150(3699):971-979.
7. Stamford JA. Descending control of pain. *Br J Anaesth.* 1995;75(2):217-227.
8. Koneru A, Satyanarayana S, Rizwan S. Endogenous opioids: their physiological role and receptors. *Global Journal of Pharmacology.* 2009;3(3):149-153.
9. Brown A. Phases of the wound healing process. *Nurs Times.* 2015;111(46)12-13.
10. Moon S, Choi J, Park S. The effects of functional electrical stimulation on muscle tone and stiffness of stroke patients. *J Phys Ther Sci.* 2017;29(2):238-241.
11. Sabut S, Sikdar C, Kumar R, Mahadevappa M. Functional electrical stimulation of dorsiflexor muscle: effects on dorsiflexor strength, plantarflexor spasticity, and motor recovery in stroke patients. *NeuroRehabilitation.* 2011;29(4):393-400. doi:10.3233/NRE-2011-0717

Thermal Agents

Chapter 3

Thermotherapy

KEY TERMS Analgesia | Conduction | Convection | Vasoconstriction | Vasodilation

CHAPTER OBJECTIVES

1. Describe the physiological effects of heat.
2. Differentiate between the methods of heat transfer.
3. Describe the importance of specific heat.
4. Categorize the indications and contraindications for thermotherapy interventions.
5. Identify when to use heat in specific clinical scenarios.
6. Document thermotherapy interventions correctly in a patient's chart.

INTRODUCTION

Heat therapy interventions transmit energy primarily via conduction and convection. Conversion, evaporation, and radiation are 3 other methods of heat transfer; these will be discussed with their specific modalities in later chapters. Conduction is the means by which heat or cold is transmitted via direct contact between a material and the tissue. For example, when one has a sore back and uses a heating pad, the heat is conducted to the tissues because it is in direct contact with the back. The same applies for a moist hot pack or when placing one's hand in a paraffin bath; because the tissue is in contact with the heating agent, the heat is transferred via conduction.

Convection relates to the movement of air, matter, or liquid around the body part. Heat is transferred to the tissues via this movement. For example, a convection oven cooks food because the heat generated inside the oven also moves around the food. With regard to modalities, fluidotherapy or a whirlpool are examples of convection.

Examples of thermal modalities in this chapter are considered superficial; that is, these modalities will not penetrate tissues greater than approximately 1 cm.[1] Thermal modalities that penetrate into deeper tissues are discussed in a later chapter. Please also remember that parameters listed in this chapter come from the available research, but parameters may vary slightly.

PHYSIOLOGICAL EFFECTS OF HEAT

To understand how and when to use heating agents for your patients, one needs to understand the physiological effects of heat on the body. This gets at the questions of "how" does the modality work? What happens in the body as a result of heat that does something useful for the patient? It is also important to note that patients are going to request the things they prefer. That is, a lot of people like heat. Even if heat is not indicated, they might request heat because it feels good.

An immediate response to heat is vasodilation, or an opening or enlargement of the blood vessels that allows

Memolo J.
Therapeutic Agents for the Physical Therapist Assistant
(pp 21-30). © 2022 SLACK Incorporated.

more blood flow to the area.[2] This yields an increased erythema, or redness. This can also increase bleeding and capillary effusion during an acute injury, which is why heat is contraindicated for acute injuries.[3] Because blood flow is increased, cooler blood can flow into the area of injury; this contrast of increased heat superficially vs the decreased heat at the site of injury can create an analgesic effect. Heat can also decrease muscle spasms, and this may provide pain relief for patients.[3] Additionally, the Gate Control theory is the working rationale for why heat decreases pain; the sensation of heat closes the gate, preventing the pain signals from being sent to the brain. This may be attributed solely to the sensory input to the Aβ fibers. There is also some research considering that increased nerve conduction may have a hand in the analgesic effects of heat.[4] Further research indicates there might be some connection with increased circulation and the removal of waste materials that could cause pain.[3]

Reflex heating, also sometimes called *consensual heat vasodilation*, is not uncommon, meaning that when heat is applied in one location, vasodilation and an increased heating of tissue remotely may occur.[5]

Increased blood flow also simulates the inflammatory process; increased amounts of oxygen, antibodies, leukocytes, and other nutrients and enzymes flood the area of injury, which can promote healing of the area. This is another reason why heat is often contraindicated for acute injuries, as it may exacerbate the signs and symptoms of inflammation. The increased blood flow can also increase localized metabolism, which allows the healing process to proceed more quickly.[3]

Heat applied to muscles and joints can increase tissue elasticity. The fluid in joints becomes less viscous (less thick) when heat is applied, allowing the joint to move more freely. Likewise, when heat is applied to musculature, the tissue becomes more extensible. This is why heat applied before or during a stretching regimen can be beneficial.[6]

While there is some evidence that muscle strength and endurance is decreased initially after the application of heat,[7] there are some studies that indicate the use of heat before exercise can reduce the development of delayed-onset muscle soreness.[8] Ultimately, heat is known to produce a relaxation effect on the muscles, but it could potentially be useful to "warm up" the tissues before activity.[3]

INDICATIONS AND CONTRAINDICATIONS OF HEAT

Indications of thermotherapy relate to its physiological effects. Because heat can increase blood flow, it should not be used for any acute injuries because this may exacerbate the inflammatory phase.[9] Subacute or chronic pain, subacute or chronic edema, or injuries are appropriate for treatment with heat. Trigger points, muscle guarding or

spasms, and decreased range of motion (ROM) are other indications of heat.

Contraindications primarily include anything that is defined as an acute injury. Additionally, if the patient has an infection, a deep vein thrombosis, areas of impaired or absent sensation, malignancies, hemorrhage, recently radiated tissues, impaired circulation, skin breakdown, or cognitive/mentation impairments, heat should generally not be applied. Pregnancy, patients with cardiac diagnoses, and areas near the eyes or carotid sinus should at least be considered precautions to heat.[9] Table 3-1 provides heat indications and contraindications as well as physiological effects.

APPLICATION METHODS

Moist Hot Packs

Commercial moist hot packs (Figure 3-1) are typically woven cotton pouches filled with bentonite, a natural hydrocolloid filling.[10] These are reusable packs that provide up to 30 minutes of moist heat at a time and come in a variety of sizes to accommodate different body sizes and body parts. The heat is conveyed via conduction. These hot packs are kept in hydrocollators that heat up water to approximately 160°F to 165°F.[11] Figure 3-2 shows one type of hydrocollator unit. There are different versions of hydrocollators out there; the traditional hydrocollators must be at higher temperatures to kill bacteria and maintain heat, but others use nonporous hot packs with gel interiors so they can be kept at lower temperatures.[12]

Traditional moist hot packs require the use of 6 to 8 layers of towels to prevent burning the patient. There are hot pack covers for the bentonite packs that count as 2 layers. Newer gel-filled versions require only 1 to 3 layers of toweling because they are stored in lower temperatures. Therapists should assess the patient's skin before treatment, as well as confirm the patient does not have any contraindications. Therapists should take care removing the hot packs from the hydrocollator, as they can be very hot. Position the patient correctly and avoid positioning the patient so they are lying on top of the hot pack because this will increase the temperature and the risk for burning. Check the patient's skin within 5 minutes of applying the hot pack and provide the patient with a bell or call light if the therapist plans to step away from the patient. If the patient complains that the hot pack is too warm, add more layers. Typical treatment times are up to 30 minutes. Discontinue the treatment if the patient's skin shows signs of burning or if the patient complains of significant pain. Table 3-2 describes the procedure for applying a moist hot pack. Figure 3-3 shows a patient receiving a hot pack treatment.

Moist hot packs, as any modality, should not be used alone; it is a tool in the physical therapist assistant's arsenal to address a patient's needs. If the patient has pain that prevents participation in therapy, heat may allay that pain

Table 3-1

Indications, Contraindications, and Physiological Effects of Heat

Indications	Contraindications	Physiological Effects
Subacute and chronic inflammation	Acute injuries	Increased superficial local temperature
Subacute edema	Impaired circulation	Increased local metabolism
Decreased ROM	Peripheral vascular disease	Vasodilation
Muscle spasm	Areas of impaired sensation or cognition	Increased blood flow
Myofascial trigger points	Deep vein thrombosis or thrombophlebitis	Increased leukocytes/phagocytosis
Subacute sprains/strains	Active hemorrhage or patients with bleeding disorders	Increased metabolic wastes
Muscle guarding	Large areas or at sufficient intensity to increase core temperature of pregnant individuals	Increased elasticity of muscles and ligaments
Delayed-onset muscle soreness	Areas of known malignancy	Analgesia
Abnormal muscle tone	Over wounds	Decreased muscle tone
Hypersensitivity	Large areas or at sufficient intensity to raise core temperature of those with severe cardiac disease/failure	Decreased muscle spasm
	Arterial disease	Increased capillary permeability
		Increased nerve conduction velocity
		Desensitization

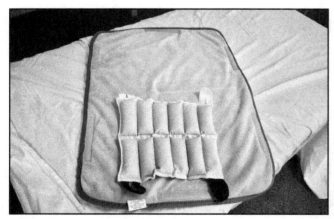

Figure 3-1. Moist hot pack (and cover).

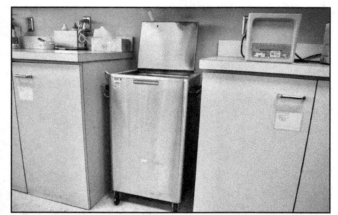

Figure 3-2. Hydrocollator unit.

long enough for the patient to participate. The American Physical Therapy Association's Choosing Wisely Campaign site also recommends that no heat modality (superficial or deep) should be used to achieve long-term outcomes.[13] While heat has been shown to provide some pain relief and can be helpful in working toward other goals, the American Physical Therapy Association states that the use of heat should be supported by evidence and "used to facilitate an active treatment program."[13]

Paraffin

A paraffin wax treatment can provide pleasant heat, similar to what one might experience in a spa treatment. Therapeutic paraffin wax has a melting point of 113°F to 121°F.[14] Paraffin wax also has a high heat capacity (but a low specific heat), which allows the patient to tolerate higher temperatures compared to the same temperature of water. Because therapeutic paraffin has mineral oil added,

Table 3-2	
Procedures for Applying Moist Hot Pack	
Equipment Needed	• Moist hot pack • Towels/hot pack covers (6 to 8 layers total) • Sheets/pillows as needed
Treatment/ Parameters	• Confirm patient does not have contraindications. • Remove jewelry, clothing, etc from treatment area and inspect skin. • Position patient for comfort and access to treatment area; drape for modesty/warmth/clothing protection. Do not allow patient to lie on top of hot pack. • Remove hot pack and place 6 to 8 layers between hot pack and tissue if using clay; 1 to 3 layers for newer packs. Secure as necessary. • Provide patient with a call bell. • Check patient's skin 5 min into treatment session. • Patient can wear hot pack for up to 20 min.
Safety Considerations	• Educate patient to use call bell if experiencing pain/burning. • Be sure to check patient's skin 5 min into treatment session; discontinue session if patient shows signs of burning.
Advantages	• Easy to use • Low level of skill required by clinician • Can cover larger areas
Disadvantages	• Must move hot pack to inspect skin • Patient may not tolerate weight of hot pack • Hot pack does not address contoured areas well • Hydrocollator and packs relatively expensive

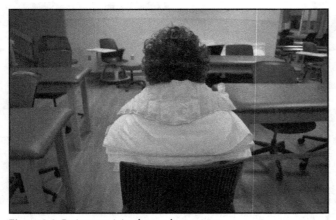

Figure 3-3. Patient receiving hot pack treatment.

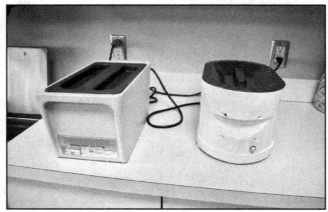

Figure 3-4. Paraffin baths (units).

it has a low melting point, making it comfortable to dip into or apply the wax to various body parts. The paraffin is kept in a thermostatically controlled container that keeps the paraffin melted for access at any time. Figure 3-4 shows examples of paraffin bath tubs. These tubs come in different sizes and are accessible from a variety of vendors. The heat is transferred via conduction.

Paraffin wax is a great option to apply heat to body parts that have grooves or contours, such as hands, feet, elbows, or knees. A study conducted in 2014 showed that paraffin wax applied to hands along with exercise was better at reducing pain than exercise alone.[15] Some clinics have special mitts or booties for hands and feet to hold in the heat; often, towels are used to wrap the body part once the wax has been applied.

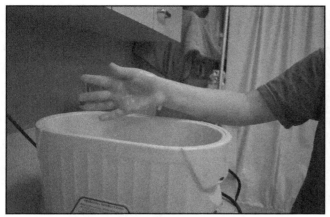

Figure 3-5. Fingers apart dipped 1 to 2 times.

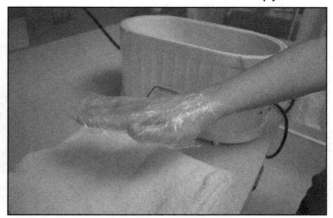

Figure 3-6. Wrapped in plastic.

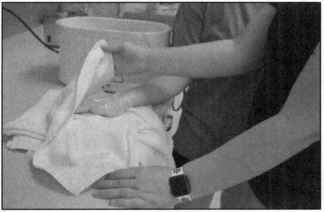

Figure 3-7. Wrapped in toweling.

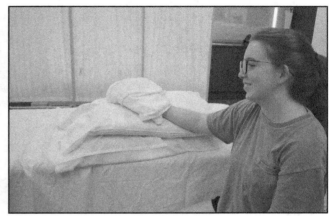

Figure 3-8. Elevated.

Before treatment, the body part should be washed and dried thoroughly. All jewelry should be removed and the skin should be inspected for open wounds, infections, or new scar tissue. There are 3 different types of application methods: the dip-wrap method, the dip-immersion method, and the paint method.

The dip-wrap method requires the patient's body part to be dipped and removed from the wax. The patient waits for the wax to solidify, and then dips and removes again, waiting a few seconds between each dip, for a total of 6 to 10 dips. After the last dip, the patient's body part is wrapped in plastic wrap and then a towel or mitt to hold in the heat. Ideally, the body part is elevated and the patient waits 10 to 15 minutes with a call bell provided in case they have pain or need assistance. Figures 3-5 through 3-8 show a patient receiving a dip-wrap treatment.

When using the dip-immersion method, the therapist dips the patient's body part initially and then removes it to allow the wax to harden. Then, the extremity is dipped again and held in the tub for the duration of the treatment, up to 20 minutes. The bath is turned off or unplugged during this treatment, and the patient is discouraged from touching the sides or bottom of the tub. The extremity is then removed and cleaned. Figure 3-9 shows a patient receiving a dip-immersion treatment.

Finally, there is the paint method, which is best for body parts that cannot be dipped directly into the tub. Wax is painted onto the body part using a paint brush. The wax should be allowed to solidify between each painted layer, for a total of 6 to 10 layers. As with the dip-wrap method, the extremity is then wrapped in plastic and a towel or mitt and elevated for 10 to 20 minutes. Figure 3-10 shows a patient receiving a paraffin paint treatment. Table 3-3 describes these methods in detail. After application of paraffin, the wax should be thrown away for infection-control purposes and the skin inspected to check for adverse effects. Patients can purchase a home paraffin wax unit as a continuation of their treatment.

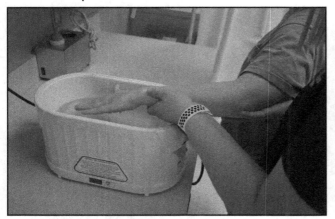

Figure 3-9. Dip-immersion method.

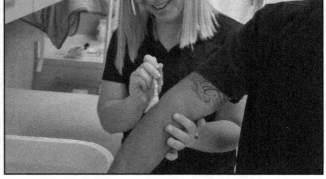

Figure 3-10. Paraffin paint method.

> ## Box 3-1
> ### Research Topic
>
> Create a research topic about fluidotherapy and its effects on patients post-stroke. Write a patient, intervention, comparison, outcome, time question and then conduct a literature review to answer your question. Think about what levels of evidence are best. What evidence is currently available? How recent is that research?

Fluidotherapy

Fluidotherapy machines distribute dry heat via convection. The machine circulates warm air and cellulose particles inside a cabinet, and a patient can put a body part inside the machine to float as if in water. Fluidotherapy machines typically run on temperatures from 100°F to 118°F.[16] Some units allow an access portal for therapists to also put in their arms and hands to provide manual therapy during the treatment. Fluidotherapy can increase superficial tissue temperature and superficial nerve conduction.[16] Physiologically, this means fluidotherapy can increase vasodilation and blood flow to the area as well as provide an analgesic effect to the area via the Gate Control theory.[4] Another physiological effect is that fluidotherapy can desensitize areas of hypersensitivity, such as in cases of complex regional pain syndrome, post-stroke, or postamputation. This is because fluidotherapy provides sensory input via the movement of air and the cellulose particles around the body part, and it is able to deliver higher temperatures comfortably. It may also affect the sensory nerve action potential conduction, which further assists in desensitization.[4] Despite these noted benefits, fluidotherapy is not a modality commonly seen in the clinic, and further research would be helpful in determining its use. See Box 3-1 for a research topic on this subject.

As with other thermal interventions, ensure the patient's skin is intact and remove any clothing or jewelry on the area to be treated. It is important to position the patient for comfort during the treatment and to secure the sleeve so the cellulose material does not escape the unit. The patient will generally receive a 20-minute treatment with the agitation level adjusted according to comfort and patient goals. The patient should also be provided a call bell in case they experience any pain or need assistance. Table 3-4 provides details of the procedure for applying fluidotherapy.

Warm Whirlpool

Whirlpool will be generally discussed here but in more detail in a later chapter as a part of hydrotherapy. Warm whirlpool distributes heat via convection when the whirlpool is on; if the water is not moving, it is considered conduction.

SAFETY CONCERNS

Patients who have contraindications should not be administered heat for their therapy interventions. Therapists should be sure to go over all possible contraindications and precautions before administering any thermotherapy.

When applying thermotherapy, the therapist should be mindful of the patient's skin condition before treatment and check the patient's skin regularly throughout the session. This is often performed visually, but if that is not possible, the therapist should consult with the patient for verbal feedback on how they are doing. This will help prevent the possibility of burning the patient, which can often be attributed to poor technique or poor patient sensation.

Even if the patient does not have contraindications or precautions, the therapist should pay attention to the patient's response to the treatment. Increased vasodilation can cause or increase bleeding; be mindful of areas that are open and bleeding (this is a contraindication) or even areas of bruising. Owing to the vasodilation, the patient may also feel lightheaded after treatment and is at a potential risk for fainting. Once the treatment is over, especially if the patient has been recumbent, let the patient sit up slowly and remain seated for a moment before getting up to ambulate.

Table 3-3
Procedures for Applying Paraffin Wax

Equipment Needed	• Paraffin wax • Plastic bags/wraps • Towels or mitts • Pillows or sheets as needed
Treatment/ Parameters	• Confirm patient does not have contraindications. • Remove jewelry, clothing, etc from treatment area and inspect the skin. • Have patient wash the body part and dry thoroughly. • Position patient for comfort and access to treatment area; drape for modesty/warmth/clothing protection. • Dip-wrap method: with fingers apart, patient dips hand into wax and remove. Let wax turn opaque and then dip again. Wait between each dip for wax to harden. Advise patient to not touch sides or bottom of bath. Dip 6 to 10 times total and then wrap with plastic bag or wrap. Follow up with a mitt or towel wrapped around body part. Advise patient to not move too much because this may break paraffin and accelerate cooling. Elevate extremity and wait 10 to 15 min or until cool. Provide patient with a call bell. • Dip-immersion method: With fingers apart, dip hand into wax and remove. Wait until wax turns opaque and dip again. Hold hand in the bath for up to 20 min, then remove. Be sure bath is turned off to prevent burning. • Paint method (ideal for body parts not easily dipped): Paint wax onto body part with a brush. Allow wax to turn opaque before applying another layer. Paint 6 to 10 layers total, waiting between each layer for wax to harden. Cover area with plastic wrap or bag and then a mitt or toweling. Advise patient to not move too much because this may break paraffin and accelerate cooling. Elevate extremity and wait 10 to 20 min or until cool. Provide patient with a call bell. • Check patient's skin after treatment session.
Safety Considerations	• Educate patient to use call bell if experiencing pain/burning.
Advantages	• Good contact with contoured areas • Easy to use • Inexpensive • Can elevate body parts during dip-wrap method • Mineral oil lubricates and conditions the skin • Can be used at home
Disadvantages	• Messy and time consuming • Cannot be used over wounds, broken skin, or new scars • Risk of contamination of wax if reused or body part not cleansed • Extremity in dependent position for dip-immersion method

	Table 3-4 Procedures for Applying Fluidotherapy			
Equipment Needed	• Fluidotherapy machine • Chair if needed			
Treatment/ Parameters	• Confirm patient does not have contraindications. • Remove jewelry, clothing, etc from treatment area and inspect skin; cover any wounds with a plastic barrier to prevent cellulose from causing further injury. • Position patient for comfort and access to treatment area; drape for modesty/ warmth/clothing protection. • Put patient's extremity through machine opening and secure sleeve to prevent cellulose from escaping. • Set temperature at 100°F to 118°F. • Agitation or air flow can be adjusted; patient should receive treatment for 15 to 20 min. • Provide patient with a call bell. • Check patient's skin after treatment session.			
Safety Considerations	• Educate patient to use call bell if experiencing pain/burning. • Ensure open wounds are covered before putting extremity in machine.			
Advantages	• Patient can move extremity inside machine during treatment • Minimal pressure applied to area • Temperature well-controlled • Easy to administer			
Disadvantages	• Expensive • Limb must be dependent • Risk of overheating			

DOCUMENTATION

This section will provide examples of documenting some thermal agents using the list of components we want to include in the "O" section of the note. The first example is of a moist hot pack treatment:

O: Patient received moist hot pack to bilateral lower lumbar spine in prone × 30 minutes with 7 layers of towels to decrease stiffness and pain. Patient was cleared of all contraindications and skin was checked after first 5 minutes of treatment with no signs of blistering or burning. Patient was provided with a call light. Patient reported the heat felt good and rated decreased pain at 3/10 after the treatment. ROM remeasured at 28 degrees extension and 45 degrees flexion.

This example addresses a paraffin treatment:

O: Patient received paraffin wax dip and wrap to right hand to address arthritic pain in the hand. Patient washed and dried hand before treatment and skin was inspected for open areas. Patient was cleared of contraindications. Patient's hand was dipped 8 times and then wrapped in plastic and covered by a towel. Patient's upper extremity was elevated and patient waited 15 minutes with call light available. After removing the wax, the patient's skin was inspected with no signs of burning or blistering. Patient reported a decrease in pain to 4/10.

CONCLUSION

Thermotherapy includes a variety of modalities, most of which are relatively inexpensive and easy to apply. Care should be given to monitor patient comfort and skin integrity, but thermotherapy is easily integrated into a patient's therapy session. Patients often enjoy thermotherapy interventions, making them excellent tools to promote function and to entice patients to participate in other therapy activities.

REVIEW QUESTIONS

1. What is the mechanism for heat transfer with a moist hot pack?
2. Describe 3 physiological effects of heat on the body.
3. How many layers should be between a patient's body and a moist hot pack?
4. Differentiate between the 3 methods to deliver a paraffin treatment.
5. What are 2 advantages of using fluidotherapy as a treatment intervention?
6. List 5 contraindications for use of thermal modalities.
7. Your patient has decreased ROM and chronic pain in their left knee. What thermal modality do you think is best for this patient? Why?
8. Your patient has tightness and pain in their upper right trapezius with decreased ROM in shoulder flexion and abduction. You want to apply a moist hot pack to this area to treat their complaints. Document your treatment including all the necessary components of an "O" section.

CASE STUDY 1

Your patient is an 18-year-old man with a lateral malleolus fracture after a soccer injury 8 weeks ago. He wore a cast for 6 weeks and a Cam boot for 2 weeks and now is in therapy to work on ROM and pain reduction. He has 11 degrees of dorsiflexion, 36 degrees of plantarflexion, 28 degrees of inversion, and 22 degrees of eversion. His fracture is completely healed, although he does complain of a dull ache, 3/10 to 4/10 pain, especially after walking for a prolonged period of time. You decide to work on improving his ROM while also addressing the patient's pain.

1. What tissues are affected?
2. What phase of healing is the patient in?
3. What thermal modality would you recommend? Why?
4. What are the physiological effects of this modality?
5. What are the contraindications of this modality?
6. Discuss the parameters of this intervention.
7. What other modality interventions (not limited to thermal) would you recommend? Why?

CASE STUDY 2

Your patient is a 67-year-old woman with rheumatoid arthritis in both hands, the left being more painful than the right. She has experienced an exacerbation of inflammation, with stiffness and a dull ache in her hands, making it difficult to garden, play with her grandchildren, or write with a pen or pencil. You would primarily like to address the patient's pain so she can resume her daily activities.

1. What are the tissues affected?
2. What modality would you select for this patient? Why?
3. What are the contraindications for this modality?
4. What are the parameters for this intervention?
5. What other intervention(s) would be appropriate? Discuss the benefits and drawbacks.

REFERENCES

1. Hawkes AR, Draper DO, Johnson AW, Diede MT, Rigby JH. Heating capacity of rebound shortwave diathermy and moist hot packs at superficial depths. *J Athl Train.* 2013;48(4):471-476.
2. Kim MY, Kim JH, Lee JU, et al. Temporal changes in pain and sensory threshold of geriatric patients after moist heat treatment. *J Phys Ther Sci.* 2011;23(5):797-801.
3. Nanneman D. Thermal modalities: heat and cold. A review of physiologic effects with clinical applications. *AAOHN J.* 1991;39(2):70-75.
4. Kelly R, Beehn C, Hansford A, Westphal KA, Halle JS, Greathouse DG. Effect of fluidotherapy on superficial radial nerve conduction and skin temperature. *J Orthop Sports Phys Ther.* 2005;35(1):16-23.
5. Mucha C. Blood flow in the forearm in patients with rheumatoid arthritis and healthy subjects under local thermotherapy. *S Afr J Physiother.* 2002;58(2):15-20.
6. Nakano J, Yamabayashi C, Scott A, Reid WD. The effect of heat with stretch to increase range of motion: a systematic review. *Phys Ther Sport.* 2012;13(3):180-188.
7. Lewis SE, Holmes PS, Woby SR, Hindle J, Fowler NE. Short term effect of superficial heat treatment on paraspinal muscle activity, stature recovery, and psychological factors in patients with chronic low back pain. *Arch Phys Med Rehabil.* 2012;93(2):367-372.
8. Petrofsky J, Berk L, Bains G, Khowailed IA, Lee H, Laymon M. The efficacy of sustained heat treatment on delayed-onset muscle soreness. *Clin J Sport Med.* 2017;27(4):329-337.
9. Electrophysical agents—contraindications and precautions: an evidence-based approach to clinical decision making in physical therapy. *Physiother Can.* 2010;62(5):1-80.
10. DJO LLC. Chattanooga Hydrocollator Hotpack set. 2019. Accessed July 25, 2019. https://www.djoglobal.com/products/chattanooga/hydrocollator-hotpac-set
11. DJO LLC. Chattanooga M-2 Mobile Heating Unit. 2019. Accessed July 25, 2019. https://www.djoglobal.com/products/chattanooga/hydrocollator-m-2-mobile-heating-unit
12. Richmar Hydratherm and Hydraheat Moist Heat Therapy System. Accessed February 2, 2022. https://static1.squarespace.com/static/5e14a119b710c24ed75fa651/t/60f18613f75f957e35bb29f2/1626441236279/1284.20.1.BMoist+HeatTherapy+Systems%5BWEB%5D.pdf

13. American Physical Therapy Association. Ten things patients and providers should question. *Choosing Wisely Campaign*. Published 2021. Accessed January 28, 2022. http://www.choosingwisely.org/societies/american-occupational-therapy-association-inc/

14. Therabath Professional Thermotherapy. Frequently asked questions. Accessed July 25, 2019. https://www.therabath.com/faq/

15. Almalty AR, Jebril M, Abu Tariah HS, Albostanji S. The effect of paraffin wax and exercise vs. exercise treatment on keyboard user's hands pain and strength. *Indian J Physiother Occup Ther*. 2014;8(1):170-175.

16. DJO LLC. Chattanooga Fluidotherapy Standard Single Extremity Unit. 2019. Accessed July 25, 2019. https://www.djoglobal.com/products/chattanooga/fluidotherapy-standard-single-extremity-unit-0

Chapter 4

Cryotherapy

KEY TERMS Analgesia | Anesthesia | Hunting response

KEY ABBREVIATIONS DOMS | DVT

CHAPTER OBJECTIVES

1. Describe the physiological effects of cold.
2. Discuss cryotherapy intervention techniques.
3. Categorize the indications and contraindications for cryotherapy interventions.
4. Identify when to use cold in specific clinical scenarios.
5. Document cryotherapy interventions correctly in a patient's chart.

INTRODUCTION

The first thing to remember when it comes to cold therapy interventions is that the effects of cold modalities are essentially the opposite of thermal modalities. That said, cold transmits energy via the same methods: conduction, convection, and evaporation. Remember that conduction transmits energy via direct contact with the energy source (eg, ice, cold packs, water). It is important to know that cold therapies do not transmit cold to the tissues; rather, cold modalities absorb heat from the tissue and lose heat to them.[1] Convection transmits energy via the movement of water or air over the body part, as in a cold whirlpool. Evaporation works the same way sweat works to cool our body; we produce sweat and as it evaporates, it produces a

cooling effect. Vapocoolant spray does the same thing in that the evaporation produces a cold effect on the tissues.

Like heat, cold is considered a superficial modality, but the depth of penetration is slightly deeper than that of superficial heat, to approximately 2 cm.[1,2] This is suggested to be due to superficial cooling that leads to the deeper tissues losing heat due to conduction (being in contact with the more superficial cooling tissues).[1] That said, cold is still considered a superficial modality, which could affect when or how a therapist plans to use cold on a patient.

PHYSIOLOGICAL EFFECTS OF COLD

As mentioned at the beginning of this chapter, an easy way to remember what cold does to the body is to remember what heat does, and then think of the opposite. For example, thermal modalities cause vasodilation and increase blood flow; in contrast, cryotherapy causes vasoconstriction and decreased blood flow.[2] As a result, any areas of hemorrhage or bruising could be affected. In addition, metabolism decreases, so in acute stages of injury cold can be useful in decreasing blood loss or swelling (which can, in turn, decrease pain). As a result, cold is often indicated immediately after an injury. A common acronym used for the treatment of an acute injury is RICE, which stands for rest, ice, compression, and elevation; this is why ice is mentioned in this acronym.

Memolo J.
Therapeutic Agents for the Physical Therapist Assistant
(pp 31-43). © 2022 SLACK Incorporated.

> ## Box 4-1
> ### Research Topic
>
> Create a patient, intervention, comparison, outcome, time question regarding the use of cryotherapy on peripheral neuropathy. What does the current research state? Are there higher level studies out there on the subject? What does your initial research tell you in response to this question?

It is worth noting that there are limits to the amount of vasoconstriction; with extensive cooling (as seen in ice immersion or ice massage), a reflex vasodilation occurs after a certain point. This is considered a protective mechanism and is sometimes called a hunting response. There is no official agreement regarding what temperature elicits such a response, although one study suggested temperatures between 5°C and 8°C (41°F to 46°F) would cause such reflexive vasodilation.[3]

Cold interventions are well known for their analgesic and anesthetic uses. Like heat, cold can decrease pain via the Gate Control theory, sending signals via the Aβ fibers to block the pain signals from the C and Aδ fibers. In addition, cold decreases nerve conduction velocity, which can slow the signals of pain to the brain. See Box 4-1 for a research topic on this subject. Unlike heat, cold can actually create an anesthetic effect to the treatment area. The common sensations a patient experiences with cryotherapy are coldness, burning, aching, and numbness; numbness can be useful to temporarily decrease or eliminate pain. Prolonged cooling of the body, especially larger portions, yields piloerection (goosebumps) and shivering, which are both ways the body strives to increase tissue temperature and blood flow. There is debate, however, as to whether cold can affect metabolism.[4]

Cold has been shown to be effective in treating myofascial pain related to trigger points as well as muscle spasms because it decreases the pain threshold and desensitizes pain receptors.[2,5,6] Cold has been shown to help with delayed-onset muscle soreness (DOMS) as a result of the nerve conduction velocity and effects of vasoconstriction, although with mixed results; ice is suggested as effective for acute muscle pain as well due to vasoconstriction.[7,8] This makes cold unique from thermotherapy interventions because it can be used both in acute and chronic conditions. This also applies to muscle and joint extensibility; although heat decreases the viscosity of joint fluid, cold increases it, making joints stiffer and not making cold a good pre-exercise or stretching modality.

Studies indicate that the temperature to which one cools the tissue and the length of time it takes to yield the positive results of cryotherapy differ for the person and body part; one must consider subcutaneous adipose tissue present in the area as well as the patient's tolerance for cold.[1] A study focusing on adipose tissue and its effects on cold indicated that the deeper the adipose tissue (measures via skin folds), the more time is required to elicit the same response with less adipose tissue.[1] There is also continued debate on the effects or usefulness of cryotherapy in treating athletes.[4]

INDICATIONS AND CONTRAINDICATIONS OF COLD

Indications for cryotherapy relate to its physiological effects. As mentioned earlier, cold causes vasoconstriction, which can be especially beneficial for acute injuries in decreasing bleeding and swelling. Owing to this and the slowed nerve conduction velocity, cold is also great for pain relief, especially if anesthesia is indicated. A study in the *International Journal of Sports Physical Therapy* indicates that ice massage may have the best initial effects for rapid anesthesia, but that the effects of ice baths or cold immersion may last longer.[4] Other indications include trigger points and muscle spasms, as well as any inflammatory process (both acute and chronic) and DOMS. This is often seen in the treatment of athletes on the sidelines of games with ice bags strapped to their shoulders or legs, or athletes may take ice baths postgame.

Just as with heat, there are certain reasons not to use cold for physical therapy interventions. Unlike heat, cold may be used both in acute and chronic conditions. However, it should not be used on patients with impaired circulation or peripheral vascular disease since cold can already decrease circulation. It should not be used on patients with cold urticaria (also known as a *cold allergy* or *intolerance*), patients with Raynaud disease (which causes some areas of the body, especially extremities, to feel numb and cold and possibly change colors in response to cold[9]), or on individuals with cryoglobulinemia (which causes abnormal proteins in the blood that clump together at temperatures below 98.6°F and impede circulation and cause skin lesions, joint pain, and peripheral neuropathy[10]). As with every modality, cryotherapy should not be used in patients with known or suspected deep vein thrombosis (DVT) or thrombophlebitis because of the risk of dislodging the clot and causing an embolism, or over areas of regenerating nerves since cold can decrease nerve conduction velocity.[11] It should be at least a precaution for applying cryotherapy on patients with decreased sensation or cognition, as they may neither feel the cold nor be able to verbalize sensations, increasing the risk for frostbite or nerve injuries.[11] Table 4-1 lists all of the indications, contraindications, and physiological effects of cryotherapy.

Table 4-1		
Indications, Contraindications, and Physiological Effects of Cold		
Indications	Contraindications	Physiological Effects
Acute pain	Persons with cold urticarial (cold allergy or hypersensitivity)	Anesthesia
Chronic pain	Individuals with Raynaud disease	Analgesia
Acute swelling	Individuals with cryoglobulinemia	Vasoconstriction
Myofascial trigger points	Impaired circulation	Hunting response
Muscle spasm	DVT or thrombophlebitis	Decreased nerve conduction velocity
Acute sprains/strains	Chronic wounds	Change in muscle strength
Acute or chronic inflammation (eg, bursitis, tendonitis)	Over-regenerating nerves	Reduction in edema
DOMS	Tissues affected by tuberculosis	Decreased localized tissue temperature
	Anterior neck/carotid sinus	
	Impaired sensation/cognition (precaution)	
	Peripheral vascular disease	

APPLICATION METHODS

Ice Bag

Also known as an *ice pack*, ice bags are exactly what they sound like: a bag filled with ice. Ideally, the bag is filled with shaved or crushed ice, as the bag will then be more malleable to the body part. The bag should be directly applied to the skin and then covered with a towel or secured in place with an elastic wrap. Figure 4-1 shows an ice bag applied to a patient. A damp towel will hold in the cold temperature better than a dry towel. Salt may be added to the ice, as this will melt the ice and further decrease the temperature. The treatment time is arguable; one study looked at 10-, 20-, and 30-minute treatment times for ice bags and determined that while all participants reported a reduction in pain and swelling, the 10-minute group demonstrated the maximal reduction of swelling and that pain reduction was not significantly different among the 3 study groups.[12] This indicates that the amount of time might be as little as 10 minutes for effective results, and the patient could reapply ice bags with 50 to 60 minutes between each treatment session.[13] Table 4-2 details the procedure for applying an ice bag.

Cold Pack

The use of a cold pack, which is a commercially produced pack kept in a refrigeration/freezer unit, is similar to that of an ice bag. Figure 4-2 shows a typical therapy freezer.

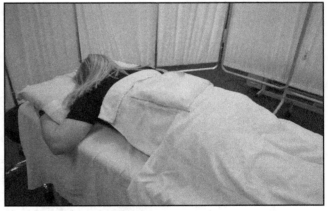

Figure 4-1. Ice bag applied to patient.

The cold packs come in a variety of sizes to accommodate different body parts (Figure 4-3) are reusable, and filled with a nontoxic silica gel, making them more pliable with respect to body parts. These packs maintain their cold temperatures for up to 30 minutes; however, it is impossible to control the temperature of a cold pack as opposed to an ice pack.[14] As with the ice bag, treatment time is not specific. One study indicated that 10- and 20-minute treatments with a cold pack can be beneficial.[15] Application can take place throughout the day every 60 to 120 minutes between each treatment session. Figure 4-4 shows the application of a cold pack to the body. Table 4-3 details the procedure for applying a cold pack to your patient.

Table 4-2
Procedures for Applying Ice Bag

Equipment Needed	• Plastic bag • Crushed/cubed ice • Towels (damp or dry) plus extra for draping • Elastic bandaging or plastic wrap • Pillows/sheets as needed
Treatment/ Parameters	• Confirm patient does not have contraindications. • Remove jewelry, clothing, etc from treatment area and inspect the skin. • Position patient for comfort and access to treatment area; drape for modesty/ warmth/clothing protection. • Place pack on skin; cover with a towel and elastic bandage/plastic wrap to decrease cold loss. • Set timer for 10 to 30 min or until patient reports numbness. Can reapply every 50 to 60 min as needed. • Provide patient with call bell. • Check patient's response verbally during treatment and check the skin after treatment session.
Safety Considerations	• Educate patient to use call bell if experiencing pain/burning.
Advantages	• Easy to use • Inexpensive • Covers moderate to large areas • Limb can be elevated • Provides more intense cooling
Disadvantages	• Must remove pack to visualize skin • Patient may not tolerate weight or wrapping of pack on limb • Pack may not contour to certain body areas

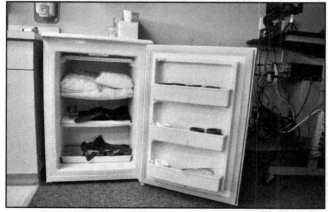

Figure 4-2. Cold pack refrigerator.

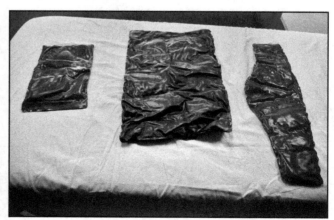

Figure 4-3. Three different-sized cold packs.

Table 4-3	
Procedures for Applying Cold Pack	
Equipment Needed	• Cold pack cooled to 8°F • Moist cold towels and dry towel plus extra for draping • Freezer unit • Elastic bandaging as needed • Pillows/sheets as needed
Treatment/ Parameters	• Confirm patient does not have contraindications. • Remove jewelry, clothing, etc from treatment area and inspect the skin. • Position patient for comfort and access to treatment area; drape for modesty/warmth/clothing protection. Elevate body part if possible. • Place wet towel on the skin and mold pack to the area; cover with a dry towel. Use elastic bandage as needed to hold pack in place. • Set timer for 10 to 20 min or until patient reports numbness. Can reapply every 1 to 2 hours as needed. • Provide patient with call bell. • Check patient's response verbally during treatment and check the skin after treatment session.
Safety Considerations	• Educate patient to use call bell if experiencing pain/burning. • Redness after treatment is normal, but rash is not.
Advantages	• Easy and quicker to apply than ice bag • Covers moderate to large areas • Limb can be elevated
Disadvantages	• Must remove pack to visualize skin • Patient may not tolerate weight or wrapping of pack on limb • Pack may not contour to certain body areas

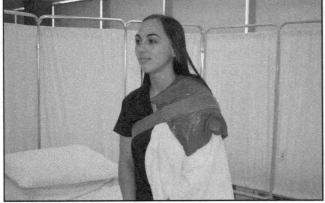

Figure 4-4. Cold pack used on patient.

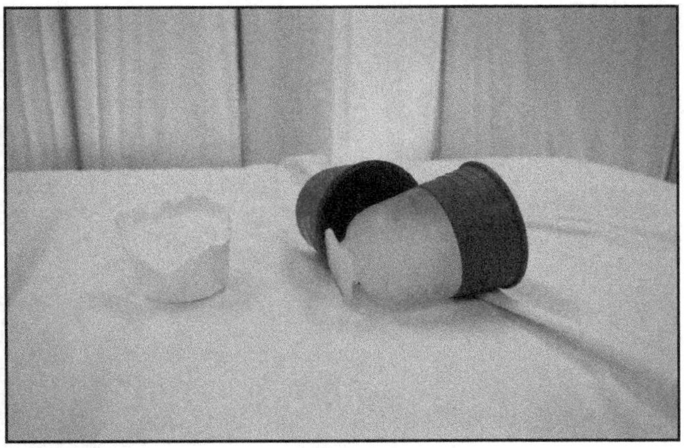

Figure 4-5. Ice massage cups (paper and plastic).

Ice Massage

Ice massage is applied by the clinician directly to the tissues. The ice can be frozen water in a paper or foam cup, or there are commercially made ice massage cups as another option (Figure 4-5). If using a paper or foam cup, the therapist will peel back the edge of paper to expose the ice; ice is applied directly to the location of pain in small circles. The patient should achieve analgesia at the site of pain, but may also reach anesthesia. Because the ice is applied directly on

	Table 4-4
	Procedures for Applying Ice Massage
Equipment Needed	• Paper or foam cup or cryocup • Freezer • Dry towels • Pillows/sheets as needed
Treatment/ Parameters	• Confirm patient does not have contraindications. • Remove jewelry, clothing, etc from treatment area and inspect the skin. • Position patient for comfort and access to treatment area; drape for modesty/warmth/clothing protection. Ideally, elevate body part if possible. • Place dry towels under and around treatment area to absorb melting water. • Apply ice directly to the tissue using small, overlapping circles. • Apply ice for 5 to 10 min or until patient reports numbness in the area. Patient will possibly report intense cold, burning, aching, and finally numbness. • Check patient's response verbally during treatment and check the skin after treatment session.
Safety Considerations	• Alert patient that redness after treatment is normal, but rash is not.
Advantages	• Easy to use • Inexpensive • Can be used for small or irregularly shaped areas • Can be applied to limb while elevated • Patient could do this at home
Disadvantages	• Time consuming for larger areas • Clinician must be present for entire treatment

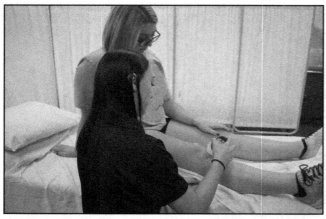

Figure 4-6. Patient receiving ice massage.

the skin, there is some thought that the effects are more intense and effective. A study comparing ice massage and ice bag determined that ice massage cooled muscle more rapidly than the ice bag.[16] Additionally, treatment time tends to be shorter than with an ice bag or cold pack. A 2015 study on pregnant women in labor determined that ice massage applied to the large intestine 4 acupressure point on the webbing of the thumb yielded decreased pain during labor.[17] Another study indicated that ice massage yields a hypoalgesic effect on study participants postexercise, meaning their sensitivity to pain was decreased.[18] Table 4-4 details how to apply ice massage, and Figure 4-6 shows a patient receiving an ice massage.

Cold Compression Unit

A later chapter will discuss the benefits and contraindications for compression, but this chapter will talk about the combination of cold and compression. Units such as an Aircast Cryo/Cuff or a Game Ready provide compression of a limb while also administering cold, and in combination they help to reduce pain as well as edema. It can be additionally beneficial in possibly preventing DVT in patients postsurgery, which is often when these units are used. One study found that in patients post–total hip arthroplasty, use of a cold compression unit resulted in less opioid use, shorter hospital stays, and less pain at 6 weeks postoperatively.[19] In an Aircast Cryo/Cuff unit (Figure 4-7) ice water is added to a cooler and the sleeve is wrapped around the

Table 4-5
Procedures for Applying Cold Compression Unit

Equipment Needed	• Cold compression unit and sleeve(s)
Treatment/ Parameters	• Confirm patient does not have contraindications. • Remove jewelry, clothing, etc from treatment area and inspect the skin. • Position patient for comfort and access to treatment area; drape for modesty/warmth/clothing protection. • Elevate area to be treated. • If it is a nondigital unit, open the valve at top of cooler. • Depending on the unit, set parameters for temperature and time, as well as if you want compression to be intermittent, If these parameters are not available, set a timer for treatment. • Patient can wear unit for 15 to 30 min every 2 hours as needed, or as recommended by patient's physician and unit manufacturer. • Check patient's response verbally during treatment and check the skin after treatment session.
Safety Considerations	• Do not apply cuff too tightly to avoid blood flow constriction. • Do not apply any other compression in addition to cuff. • Ensure patient has call bell if left unattended.
Advantages	• Allows simultaneous application of cold and compression • Temperature and compression can be controlled (in some units) • Can be applied to large joints
Disadvantages	• Units can be expensive • Treatment is available only for extremities • Treatment site cannot be visualized during treatment session • Difficult to control temperature and compression force

body part.[20] Ideally, the limb is also elevated to additionally reduce swelling. Cold water will travel via a tube from the cooler to the sleeve; there are different sleeves for different body parts. The sleeve should be empty of water before application, so the tube will be connected to the sleeve after applying the sleeve. The physical therapist assistant must then raise the cooler to allow water to filter down into the sleeve and then place the cooler on level with the sleeve. Some versions plug in and provide intermittent compression. A Game Ready is similar in that it is a machine connected to a sleeve that wraps the affected limb or area. It circulates cold water and provides intermittent compression at the same time; it differs from the Cryo/Cuff in that it is a "higher-tech" machine (and also more costly) with adjustable compression levels and a timer.[21] There are other brand-name devices that perform the same task, and it will depend on the manufacturer's recommendations exactly how to apply as well as how long to wear the modality. Table 4-5 details the procedure for applying a cold compression unit.

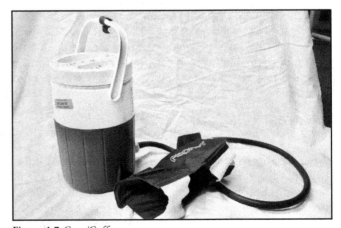

Figure 4-7. Cryo/Cuff.

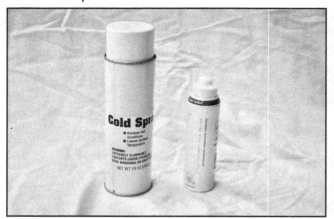

Figure 4-8. Vapocoolant spray.

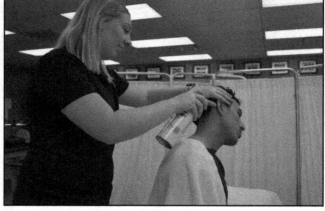

Figure 4-9. Vapocoolant spray with stretch.

Vapocoolant Spray

There are a variety of vapocoolant spray brands, and each has its own application procedures. The chemicals used may also vary; the vapocoolant spray produced by the Gebauer Company includes pentafluoropropane and tetrafluoroethane,[22] while others include ethyl chloride.[23] While the other cryotherapy methods discussed so far cool the body via conduction, vapocoolant spray cools via evaporation, much like sweat, when it dries on the skin, it cools the body. Figure 4-8 shows examples of vapocoolant spray. Application requires the can to be held upright and anywhere from 3 to 18 inches away from the skin, depending on the manufacturer's recommendations and treatment goals. Gebauer Company's recommendations are to hold the can 3 to 7 inches away for topical anesthesia, whereas 12 to 18 inches is more appropriate for stretching.[24] Ideally, the body part being sprayed is put in a position of stretch and that positioning is held in the position after spraying if doing so for myofascial pain; spray should be in parallel lines following the direction of the tissue (Figure 4-9). Avoid spraying back and forth. A 2016 study showed that use of vapocoolant spray before venipuncture decreased pain significantly with minor adverse effects.[25] Table 4-6 lists the steps for applying vapocoolant spray to your patient.

Contrast Bath

It is known that heat causes vasodilation, whereas cold causes vasoconstriction (to a degree). What happens, then, if you put the 2 together? Contrast baths have been used in the clinic as a means to gain the benefits of both hot and cold therapies, such as pain control. It is also widely believed that contrast baths increase or improve circulation[26] or can help reduce swelling, as the vasoconstriction. and vasodilation produce a pumping effect on the circulatory system.

In a contrast bath set-up, 2 containers are filled with water. One holds cold water (50°F to 60°F) and the other is filled with hot water (100°F to 110°F).[27] The patient is then positioned so they can dip the affected body part into the tubs of water and alternate back and forth. There are conflicting studies on the ratio of hot to cold alterations. The standard recommendation is to have 3 to 5 cycles of a 3:1 or 4:1 hot to cold ratio. However, one study compared a 3:1 hot to cold ratio performed 3 times to an initial 3:1 ratio and then a 10-minute dip in warm water only for the second (and final) cycle.[28] The study determined that participants' artery mean blood velocity (aMBV) increased in the first cycles of both study groups; however, in the group with the second 10-minute heating-only cycle, participants' aMBV percentages increased.[28] Their conclusion was that a longer heating time in second or third cycles would be more beneficial than the standard 3:1 ratio recommendation. Some therapists choose to start and end with the hot water; other therapists opt to end with the cold water. There is no specific evidence that one method is better than the other. Table 4-7 lists the procedure for applying a contrast bath. See also Box 4-2 for a research topic on contrast baths.

Ice Immersion

Earlier it was mentioned that athletes often submerge body parts or their entire bodies in ice baths postgame. Ice immersion is often used as a technique to reduce swelling, and many use it as a method to reduce the severity of DOMS. One study showed that 10 minutes of ice immersion at 50°F reduced DOMS and improved joint range of motion (ROM) in participants 48 hours after exercise.[29] The temperature of the water varies according to sources, but it ranges from 50°F to 60°F; the time of treatment also varies, as some studies have participants immerse for 3 minutes and others up to 20 minutes. A 2016 systematic review that aimed to determine what temperatures and immersion time provide the best outcomes determined that temperatures between 50°F and 64°F and treatment times of 10 to 20 minutes yielded the best results.[30] The lower the temperature used, the less time is required to achieve numbness. Often treatment time is listed as being until the patient reports numbness in that area. Table 4-8 lists the steps for treating your patient with ice immersion.

Table 4-6 Procedures for Applying Vapocoolant Spray	
Equipment Needed	• Vapocoolant spray • Towel to drape patient
Treatment/ Parameters	• Confirm patient does not have contraindications. • Remove jewelry, clothing, etc from treatment area and inspect the skin. • Position patient for comfort and access to treatment area; drape for modesty/ warmth/clothing protection. If spraying near patient's face, drape to prevent inhalation or injury to eyes/face. • Passively position treatment site on stretch if treating for trigger point or myofascial pain. • Follow manufacturer's recommendations; holding can upright, hold can ~ 3 to 7 inches away and spray for 4 to 10 seconds for topical anesthesia. If addressing myofascial pain, position tissue on passive stretch, hold can at 30-degree angle, and hold can 12 to 18 inches away from skin. Make parallel sweeps of spray in one direction following direction of the muscle until entire muscle is covered. Maintain or increase stretch after spraying and repeat as needed. • If stretching, rewarm tissues after treatment via moist heat 10 to 15 min. • Check patient's response verbally during treatment and check the skin after treatment session.
Safety Considerations	• Patient and therapist should not inhale vapors from spray; ensure patient is draped accordingly.
Advantages	• Brief treatment time • Localized treatment area • Relatively inexpensive • Effective for trigger points
Disadvantages	• Limited to brief, localized, and superficial cold treatment • Difficult to control spray • Risk of frostbite if tissue is not rewarmed between treatments

Cold Whirlpool

As with the warm whirlpool, more will be mentioned in a later chapter. Heat is transferred via conduction when the water is in contact with the body and via convection when the water is moving. Table 4-9 describes how to apply a cold whirlpool.

SAFETY CONCERNS

Safety considerations for patients receiving cryotherapy are similar to those of thermotherapy. The therapist should be aware of all contraindications and avoid treating patients with those limitations. Even if the patient does not have specific contraindications, be mindful of the patient's status is they have diabetes, neuropathy, or other circulation or sensation impairments. Because cryotherapy typically transfers energy via conduction, one must monitor a patient's skin carefully before, during, and after treatment. Be sure to ask the patient for verbal feedback regarding the treatment intervention and make adjustments to the treatment if the patient verbalizes discomfort or pain.

DOCUMENTATION

The following shows documentation for a cold pack application for left wrist pain.

O: Patient is seated with left upper extremity supported on a wedge with a cold pack applied over a wet towel × 10 minutes to left dorsal wrist. The patient reported feeling numb at the end of the treatment with a pain rating of 3/10. Skin inspection post treatment showed some redness in the area but no other concerns.

	Table 4-7
	Procedures for Applying Contrast Bath
Equipment Needed	• Two containers; whirlpools can be used if needed • Ice • Access to warm/hot water • Towels • Chair (possibly)
Treatment/ Parameters	• Confirm patient does not have contraindications. • Remove jewelry, clothing, etc from treatment area and inspect the skin. • Position patient for comfort and access to treatment area; drape for modesty/ warmth/clothing protection. • Fill 2 tubs or whirlpools with water. Warm water (100°F to 110°F) and cold water (50°F to 60°F). • Have patient alternate dipping extremity into hot and cold water, starting in warm. A 3:1 or 4:1 ratio is standard; more effects have been noted with initial 3:1 ratio the first cycle and a 7:1 to 10:1 ratio subsequent times. A total of 3 to 5 cycles, or up to 30 min, is standard. • Check patient's response verbally during treatment and check the skin after treatment session.
Safety Considerations	• Be mindful that the hot water is not too hot for patient tolerance or safety.
Advantages	• Relatively inexpensive • Provides good contact with contoured areas • Allows freedom of movement in the water during treatment session
Disadvantages	• Therapist must maintain the water temperatures throughout the session • Patient's extremity cannot be elevated during treatment • This method requires a relatively large area • It is messy • It may require therapist to stay close by if patient is unable to alternate according to time independently

Box 4-2

Research Topic

Create a patient, intervention, comparison, outcome, time question regarding the use of contrast baths on blood flow—specifically, look at its use in patients with and without diabetes. What does the research say on this topic? How recent is the research, and what is missing?

The next example describes how a cold compression unit treatment to the right knee would be documented.

O: Patient in supine with bolster under right knee. Applied cryocuff to right knee and timer set for 20 minutes. Patient was draped with sheet to maintain warmth and comfort during the treatment session. Patient reported no discomfort and a decrease of pain to a 4/10.

CONCLUSION

While some patients prefer heat to cold, cryotherapy offers many benefits over heat for specific patient diagnoses. It is especially beneficial for acute or subacute injuries and is able to provide anesthesia in addition to analgesia. Be sure to ask the patient for feedback regarding sensations and check the patient's skin after the treatment session. Cold is relatively easy and inexpensive to add to a treatment session, and some patients prefer the pain relief it offers after a taxing therapy session.

Table 4-8
Procedures for Applying Ice Immersion

Equipment Needed	• Tub or container • Ice water • Towels
Treatment/ Parameters	• Confirm patient does not have contraindications. • Remove jewelry, clothing, etc from treatment area and inspect the skin. • Position patient for comfort and access to treatment area; drape for modesty/ warmth/clothing protection. • Place dry towels under and around treatment area to absorb melting water. • Have patient immerse body part into ice bath (50°F to 64°F) for 10 to 20 min or until area is numb. • Check patient's response verbally during treatment and check the skin after treatment session.
Safety Considerations	• Alert patient that redness after treatment is normal. • Coldness pain may be significant.
Advantages	• Easy to use • Can be used at home • Relatively inexpensive • Contours to irregularly shaped areas
Disadvantages	• Messy • Patient's body part must be in dependent position • Patient may find treatment uncomfortable

REVIEW QUESTIONS

1. How does cold transfer heat from patients?
2. List 5 physiological effects of cold.
3. What are the treatment parameters for vapocoolant spray? How would you document this?
4. Name 3 indications and 3 contraindications for cryotherapy interventions.
5. Your patient has come to the therapy clinic complaining of pain in their left elbow. After talking with the patient, the physical therapist discovers that the patient injured their elbow yesterday when lifting a box of books. Is their injury appropriate for cryotherapy interventions (based on this information)? Why or why not?
6. You saw a patient for pain in their patellar tendon and you want to apply ice therapy. Document the "O" section of your treatment session with this patient.
7. Your patient comes in with pain in their left ankle after rolling it 4 days ago during a soccer match. The pain is accompanied by swelling. What cryotherapy intervention do you think would be best and why?
8. What are 2 advantages and 3 disadvantages of cold immersion?

CASE STUDY 1

Your patient is a 38-year-old woman who complains of 7/10 pain in her elbow, especially when she lifts grocery bags or her baby carrier. The referring physician has diagnosed her with medial epicondylitis, and the physical therapist would like you to work on decreasing pain while improving mobility and function.

1. What tissues are injured/affected?
2. What cryotherapy modality would you select for this patient? Why?
3. What are the physiological effects of this intervention?
4. What are the contraindications?
5. What are the parameters for this intervention?
6. What other modality would you select for this patient (does not have to be cryotherapy)? Why?

Table 4-9 Procedures for Applying Cold Whirlpool	
Equipment Needed	• Access to cold water • Whirlpool tank with turbine • Heated, well-ventilated space • (Heated) towels
Treatment/ Parameters	• Confirm patient does not have contraindications. • Remove jewelry, clothing, etc from treatment area and inspect the skin. • Position patient for comfort and access to treatment area; drape for modesty/warmth/clothing protection. • Have towels ready to wipe up excess water once modality is complete. • Fill the tank with water of appropriate temperature. • Position patient for comfort/access; drape for modesty/warmth/clothing protection. Make sure there is no pressure on limb that is submerged. If patient has wound dressing, remove before treatment. No clothing should be in the tank because it can get tangled in the turbine. • Direct turbine to either point at or away from treatment area. • Turn on unit; stay with patient during the session and monitor response. • Check patient's response verbally during treatment and check the skin after treatment session. • Clean up after treatment; wipe down whirlpool according to directions provided. • Typically applied 10 to 30 min depending on treatment goal.
Safety Considerations	• Monitor for patient pain. • If patient is bleeding during treatment, will need to stop treatment. • Monitor patient vital signs and discontinue if they stray from normal. • Patient might be chilled or lightheaded after treatment.
Advantages	• Patient can be positioned comfortably during treatment • Allows for movement of extremity during treatment
Disadvantages	• Size of tank requires large quantity of water • Risk of infection transmission if not cleaned properly • Time to fill and clean tank as well as prepare patient

CASE STUDY 2

Your patient, a 52-year-old man, fell on the ice outside his house when retrieving the mail and sustained a Colles fracture of his left wrist 10 weeks ago. After surgery, he wore a cast for 8 weeks and has been wearing a brace since having the cast removed to support the wrist. He reports the wrist feels stiff and is at times painful, but he is eager to use it more since he is left handed. Wrist flexion is 72 degrees, extension is 48 degrees, ulnar deviation is 28 degrees, and radial deviation is 18 degrees. Your goal is to improve his ROM while also limiting his pain.

1. What tissues were injured?
2. What phase of healing is this patient in?
3. What is the cryotherapy intervention you would recommend? Why?
4. Discuss the physiological method for reducing pain that this intervention uses.
5. What are the parameters for this intervention?
6. What other interventions would you recommend (not necessarily cryotherapy)? Why?

REFERENCES

1. Merrick MA, Jutte LS, Smith ME. Cold modalities with different thermodynamic properties produce different surface and intramuscular temperatures. *J Athl Train.* 2003;38(1):28-33.

2. Nanneman D. Thermal modalities: heat and cold. A review of physiologic effects with clinical applications. *AAOHN J.* 1991;39(2):70-75.

3. Mekjavic IB, Dobnikar U, Kounalakis SN. Cold-induced vasodilation response in the fingers at 4 different water temperatures. *Appl Physiol Nutr Metab.* 2013;38(1):14-20.

4. Hawkins SW, Hawkins JR. Clinical applications of cryotherapy among sports physical therapists. *Int J Sports Phys Ther.* 2016;11(1):141-148.

5. Rajarajeswaran P. Effects of spray and stretch technique and post isometric relaxation technique in acute active central trigger point of upper trapezius. *Indian J Physiother Occup Ther.* 2010;4(4):121-124.

6. Algafly AA, George KP. The effect of cryotherapy on nerve conduction velocity, pain threshold and pain tolerance. *Br J Sports Med.* 2007;41(6):365-369.

7. Torres R, Ribeiro F, Duarte JA, Cabri JMH. Evidence of the physiotherapeutic interventions used currently after exercise-induced muscle damage: systematic review and meta-analysis. *Phys Ther Sport.* 2012;13(2):101-114.

8. Burgess T, Lambert M. The efficacy of cryotherapy on recovery following exercise-induced muscle damage. *ISMJ.* 2010;11(2):258-277.

9. Mayo Clinic. Raynaud's disease. 2019. Accessed September 12, 2019. https://www.mayoclinic.org/diseases-conditions/raynauds-disease/symptoms-causes/syc-20363571

10. Mayo Clinic. Cryoglobulinemia overview. 2019. Accessed September 12, 2019. https://www.mayoclinic.org/diseases-conditions/cryoglobulinemia/symptoms-causes/syc-20371244

11. Electrophysical agents—contraindications and precautions: an evidence-based approach to clinical decision making in physical therapy. *Physiother Can.* 2010;62(5):1-80.

12. Kuo CC, Lin CC, Lee WJ, Huang WT. Comparing the antiswelling and analgesic effects of three different ice pack therapy durations: a randomized controlled trial on cases with soft tissue injuries. *J Nurs Res.* 2013;21(3):186-193.

13. Fang L, Hung CH, Wu SL, Fang SH, Stocker J. The effects of cryotherapy in relieving postarthroscopy pain. *J Clin Nurs.* 2011;21(5-6):636-643.

14. DJO. Chattanooga ColPac Cold Therapy. 2019. September 12, 2019. https://www.djoglobal.com/products/chattanooga/colpac-cold-therapy

15. Kostaki A, Fousekis M, Larsen K. The effect of local cold pack application for 10 and 20 minutes on active and passive hamstrings flexibility in collegiate soccer players. *Physiotherapy Issues.* 2012;8(3):67-76.

16. Zemke JE, Andersen JC, Guion WK, McMillan J, Joyner AB. Intramuscular temperature responses in the human leg to two forms of cryotherapy: ice massage and ice bag. *J Orthop Sports Phys Ther.* 1998;27(4):301-307.

17. Kamali S, Jafari E, Tehran HA, Mazloomzadeh S. The effect of ice massage of the LI4 point on severity of labor pain in primigravidas. *Qom Univ Med Sci J.* 2015;8(6):61-65.

18. Anaya-Terroba L, Arroyo-Morales M, Fernández-de-Las-Peñas C, Díaz-Rodríguez L, Cleland JA. Effects of ice massage on pressure pain thresholds and electromyography activity postexercise: a randomized controlled crossover study. *J Manipulative Physiol Ther.* 2010;33(3):212-219.

19. Leegwater NC, Willems JH, Brohet R, Nolte PA. Cryocompression therapy after elective arthroplasty of the hip. *Hip Int.* 2012;22(5):527-533.

20. DJO Global. Aircast Cryo/Cuff. 2019. Accessed September 26, 2019. https://www.djoglobal.com/products/aircast/cryocuff-ic-cooler

21. Game Ready. GRPRO 2.1. 2019. Accessed September 26, 2019. https://gameready.com/gr-pro-cold-therapy-unit/

22. Gebauer Company. Safety data sheet: Gebauer's Spray and Stretch. 2013. Accessed September 26, 2019. https://cdn2.hubspot.net/hubfs/150313/docs/Spray_and_Strech/Safety_Sheet/SS_English_SDS.pdf

23. Vidant Pharma Ltd. Safety data sheet: Ethyl Chloride Vidant Pharma Spray/Stream. 2015. Accessed September 26, 2019. https://www.medguard.ie/amfile/file/download/file_id/1634/product_id/13335/

24. Gebauer Company. Gebauer's Spray and Stretch product information. 2018. Accessed September 26, 2019. https://cdn2.hubspot.net/hubfs/150313/Spray%20and%20Stretch%20Product%20Information.pdf

25. Mace SE. Prospective, randomized, double-blind controlled trial comparing vapocoolant spray vs placebo spray in adults undergoing venipuncture. *Am J Emerg Med.* 2016;34(5):798-804.

26. Shadgan B, Pakravan AH, Hoens A, Reid WD. Contrast baths, intramuscular hemodynamics, and oxygenation as monitored by near-infrared spectroscopy. *J Athl Train.* 2018;53(8):782-787.

27. Cincinnati Children's Hospital. 1987. Home instructions for contrast bath. Accessed February 2, 2022. https://www.cincinnatichildrens.org/-/media/cincinnati%20childrens/home/service/r/rheumatology/patients/home/home-contrast-bath.pdf?la=en

28. Shih CY, Lee WL, Lee CW, Huang CH, Wu YZ. Effect of time ratio of heat to cold on brachial artery blood velocity during contrast baths. *Phys Ther.* 2012;92(3):448-453.

29. Lynch E, Barry S. The effectiveness of ice water immersion in the treatment of delayed onset muscle soreness in the lower leg. *Physiother Pract Res.* 2012;33(1):9-15.

30. Machado AF, Ferreira PH, Micheletti JK, et al. Can water temperature and immersion time influence the effect of cold water immersion on muscle soreness? A systematic review and meta-analysis. *Sports Med.* 2016;46(4):503-514.

Unit III

Sound-Energy Modalities

Chapter 5

Therapeutic Ultrasound and Phonophoresis

KEY TERMS Acoustic streaming | Attenuation | Beam nonuniformity rate | Cavitation | Continuous | Duty cycle | Effective radiating area | Frequency | Microstreaming | Piezoelectric | Pulsed | Reflection | Refraction | Spatial average temporal average intensity | Spatial average temporal peak intensity

KEY ABBREVIATIONS BNR | ERA | SATA | SATP | W/cm^2

CHAPTER OBJECTIVES

1. Compare thermal and nonthermal physiological effects of ultrasound.
2. Describe the physiological effects and purpose of applying phonophoresis.
3. Discuss ultrasound intervention techniques.
4. Categorize the indications and contraindications for ultrasound interventions.
5. Apply knowledge of ultrasound/phonophoresis parameters to case scenarios.
6. Document ultrasound/phonophoresis interventions correctly in a patient's chart.

INTRODUCTION

Patients often misunderstand when told they are to receive an ultrasound treatment; they may think about the type of ultrasound used to view inside the body. Although therapeutic ultrasound works off similar principles as diagnostic ultrasound, the frequency used differs, as do the outcomes. Ultrasound is a type of sound wave (like ultraviolet light is a type of light), but it has a frequency much higher than what the human ear can detect, which is 20,000 cycles/second or hertz (Hz). By comparison, ultrasound is measured in megahertz (MHz), which is millions of cycles/second. Similar to how the sound of a fire engine siren grows quieter the farther away it is, the intensity of ultrasound energy decreases as it passes through material, which is called *attenuation*. Energy is transmitted via conversion, meaning the sound energy is converted into heat.

As an ultrasound wave enters a tissue, it can be absorbed, reflected, or refracted. Absorbed ultrasound yields heat. Reflected ultrasound bounces off a surface and is redirected in an equal and opposite angle away from that surface, such as when ultrasound hits bone. Reflection also occurs when ultrasound hits air, which will be an important factor to discuss during the parameters and application portion of this chapter. Refraction is when the ultrasound enters the tissue and is redirected at another angle but still in the tissue. Think of viewing a straw in a glass of water from the side; the straw looks bent because the light through the water has refracted the image (Figure 5-1).

An ultrasound machine has a transducer, or sound head, to administer the ultrasound waves to the tissue. Ultrasound heads come in a variety of sizes, and one should select the size according to the body part being treated. Figure 5-2 shows different sound head sizes. Inside this transducer is a piezoelectric crystal that responds to the alternating electrical current sent from the machine. The electrical current causes the crystal to expand and contract, causing an ultrasound wave. The crystal in the transducer is fragile, so care is needed when handling the sound head.

Memolo J.
Therapeutic Agents for the Physical Therapist Assistant
(pp 47-56). © 2022 SLACK Incorporated.

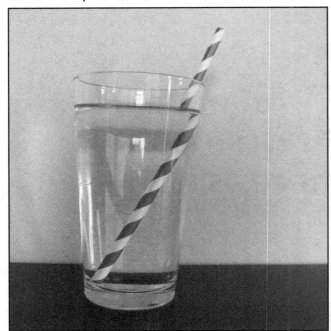

Figure 5-1. Glass with straw (refracted image).

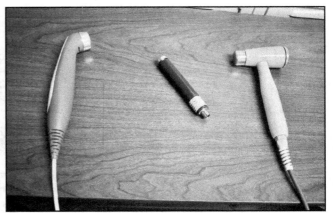

Figure 5-2. Ultrasound heads in a variety of sizes.

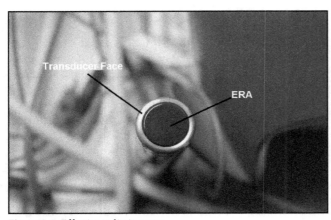

Figure 5-3. Effective radiating area.

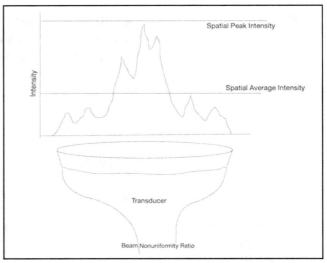

Figure 5-4. BNR with spike.

Additionally, because ultrasound cannot travel through air, the unit should not be on unless the sound head is in contact with a coupling medium and the tissue being treated.

Providing a safe ultrasound treatment means knowing the effective radiating area (ERA) of the transducer. This is the area of the sound head that actually produces ultrasound energy, and it is ideally almost identical to, but is typically slightly smaller than, the diameter of the sound head itself (Figure 5-3). Therefore, one should treat an area only 2 to 3 times the size of the ERA of the sound head or 2 times the size of the sound head.[1] This limits the ultrasound treatment to relatively small areas. A larger area with ultrasound can be treated, but one would have to perform several ultrasound treatments (rather than one longer treatment) to affect the entire area.

An ultrasound beam is variable in the intensity of energy delivered; this is called *beam nonuniformity ratio*. The ratio is determined by measuring the peak intensity from the sound head as it compares to the average output of ultrasound from the sound head. The ratio should be 1:1; however, 2:1 up to 6:1 is more common. The lower this ratio, the more uniform the beam across the sound head and the less likely one will experience a hot spot during treatment. Figure 5-4 provides an example of the beam nonuniformity ratio on a sound head.

Therapeutic ultrasound can be used for a variety of purposes, which will be discussed later in this chapter. Figures 5-5 through 5-7 show a variety of ultrasound units. Phonophoresis, or the use of ultrasound to deliver topical medications, will also be discussed in this chapter, including the medications that can be delivered and the parameters used for this intervention. The therapist using therapeutic ultrasound should know how to set ultrasound parameters to address specific tissues and diagnoses, but first, the therapist needs to understand how ultrasound works.

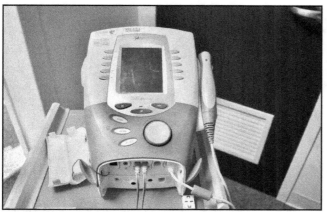

Figure 5-5. Ultrasound unit.

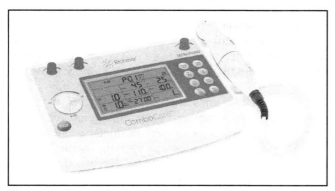

Figure 5-7. Ultrasound unit.

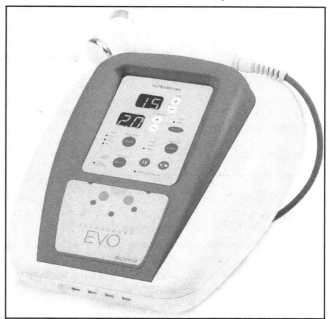

Figure 5-6. Ultrasound unit.

PHYSIOLOGICAL EFFECTS OF ULTRASOUND

Thermal Effects

Ultrasound can be categorized as being thermal or nonthermal; another way to look at it is that the ultrasound is being distributed in a continuous or pulsed mode. If the ultrasound wave is on continuously, a thermal effect is generated and both deep and superficial tissues can be heated. The type of tissue being treated can affect the amount of heating that occurs. Tissues with a high collagen content, such as tendons, ligaments, fascia, muscle, or joint capsules, heat faster than those with a low collagen content (which often have a high water content).

When ultrasound generates thermal effects, it is said to be on a continuous duty cycle. The duty cycle is one of the parameters set when providing an ultrasound treatment, and it is the percentage of time the ultrasound is on. A continuous duty cycle is on 100% of the time (or the duty cycle is 100%), and because it is on 100% of the time, the ultrasound will generate heat.

Because continuous (or thermal) ultrasound generates heat, the physiological effects (and thus the indications)

are similar to those of any other thermal modality. These include an increase in tissue extensibility, a decrease of joint stiffness, a reduction of muscle spasms, increased blood flow due to vasodilation, and an overall reduction in pain. Ultrasound can penetrate deeper than other thermotherapy interventions, so it is ideal to target deeper tissues.

Something to keep in mind when using thermal ultrasound to promote stretching of soft tissue is to put the area being treated in a stretched position during the ultrasound treatment and maintain that stretch for several minutes after the treatment is completed. This will increase the likelihood of the stretch being effective and longer-lasting.

Nonthermal Effects

If the ultrasound is on a pulsed mode (meaning the ultrasound turns on and off), the effect is nonthermal. A pulsed duty cycle is anything that is not on 100% of the time, and options can include a 10%, 20%, or 50% duty cycle. A 20% duty cycle means the ultrasound output is on 20% of the time, and the time the ultrasound is off allows heat to disperse without sufficiently heating the tissues.

While continuous ultrasound generates thermal effects similar to those generated with thermotherapy, nonthermal ultrasound's effects include acoustic streaming, which is the circular flow of cellular fluids; microstreaming, which is the small eddying that occurs around any vibrating object; and cavitation, which is the formation of gas-filled bubbles as a result of ultrasound energy. Through the process of rarefaction, these bubbles expand and then shrink during compression. Cavitation can be stable, during which time the bubbles oscillate but do not burst. Stable cavitation is thought to be what generates the therapeutic effects of

Box 5-1

Research Topic

Conduct some research on the use of therapeutic ultrasound to aid in bone healing. What do you find? Is the research current? A higher level of evidence? Now conduct some research on the use of ultrasound to treat plantar fasciitis. What does the research say about its use for this diagnosis? What do you notice about the research out there on these subjects?

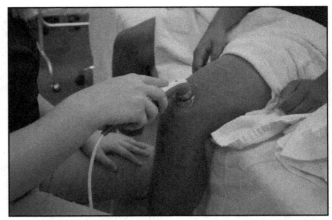

Figure 5-8. Ultrasound applied to knee.

nonthermal ultrasound. Cavitation can also be unstable, causing the bubbles to grow and implode. The results of these implosions are not therapeutic, and can generate temporary increases in heat as well as free radical formation. Acoustic streaming, microstreaming, and cavitation alter a membrane or tissue's permeability.

As a result of these effects, nonthermal (pulsed) ultrasound is often used for tissue healing. This could apply to wound healing[2] as well as tendon/ligament or even bone fracture healing.[3] The idea is that pulsed ultrasound promotes osteoblast and fibroblast proliferation, as well as promoting collagen synthesis and affecting the proteins related to bone growth.[4]

INDICATIONS AND CONTRAINDICATIONS OF ULTRASOUND

The indications for ultrasound include indications similar to those of thermal modalities, but they also include additional diagnoses related to the nonthermal effects ultrasound can produce. Indications include pain, wounds, bone fractures, soft-tissue injuries, inflammation, and acute as well as subacute or chronic conditions. See Box 5-1 for a research topic on the uses of therapeutic ultrasound. Figure 5-8 shows a patient receiving ultrasound to the knee.

Contraindications include avoiding thermal ultrasound for acute or subacute injuries, avoiding the use of ultrasound over malignancies or infections, and avoiding its use over a pregnant patient's abdomen, low back, or pelvis. Ultrasound can increase circulation and thus promote the spread of a cancer or infection to other areas, and the effects of heat could potentially cause birth defects. Another contraindication includes using ultrasound over central nervous system tissue because it could damage the tissue. Therefore, when applying a treatment to the low back, one would not use ultrasound over the spinal cord area but would instead perform 2 separate treatments on each side of the back. One should not apply ultrasound over areas with joint cement or plastic; the vibrations could loosen the connection with cement or overly heat the plastic. Ultrasound may be appropriate to use over metal implants, screws, or plates, as it has not been shown to overheat or loosen metal in some studies.[5] Do not use ultrasound over the area of a pacemaker, but it can be used distal to that area. It should not be applied to patients with thrombophlebitis or deep vein thrombosis so as to not dislodge a clot and cause an embolus.

Additional contraindications include not applying ultrasound over the eyes, reproductive organs, epiphyseal plates (in growing children), or over breast implants. The effects of cavitation and heat could impair vision, negatively affect gamete development, change bone growth, or rupture implants. Table 5-1 includes a list of ultrasound indications, contraindications, and physiological effects.

APPLICATION METHODS

Ultrasound has 4 main parameters to set when deciding on a treatment protocol for a patient. Parameters are decided based on the desire to heat or not heat tissues, the depth of tissue being targeted, the patient's level of comfort during the treatment, and the size of the treatment area.

Duty cycle was already discussed previously as a factor affecting whether ultrasound produces thermal or nonthermal effects. The duty cycle should be set according to the clinician's goal; if the aim is to stretch tissue or provide pain relief, a 100% duty cycle is required. However, if the goal is to heal tissue or address an inflammatory response during the acute phase of healing, a nonthermal duty cycle of 10%, 20%, or 50% is necessary.

Ultrasound frequency is another parameter set during an ultrasound treatment. The depth of penetration (and thus, a factor in what tissue is heated) is determined by the ultrasound frequency. Most ultrasound units offer a 1-MHz or 3-MHz frequency; 3 MHz penetrates less than 2.5 cm, whereas 1 MHz penetrates 2.5 to 5 cm.[6] The 3-MHz frequency is also absorbed faster than the 1-MHz frequency.[6] Select the frequency based on the tissue targeted; a more superficial area will require 3 MHz, and 1 MHz is more appropriate for deeper tissues.

Table 5-1
Indications, Contraindications, and Physiological Effects of Ultrasound

Indications	Contraindications	Physiological Effects
Acute pain (nonthermal)	Impaired circulation	Gate Control theory (pain; thermal and nonthermal)
Chronic pain (thermal)	Eyes, anterior neck, carotid sinus, reproductive organs	Vasodilation (thermal)
Chronic inflammation (thermal)	Deep vein thrombosis or thrombophlebitis	Increased blood flow (thermal)
Myofascial trigger points (thermal or nonthermal)	Malignancy (local)	Increased elasticity of muscles/tissues (thermal)
Muscle spasm (thermal)	Pregnancy (local)	Decreased muscle spasm (thermal)
Sprains/strains (thermal or nonthermal depending on acuteness)	Plastic or cemented implants (local)	Cavitation (nonthermal)
Soft-tissue healing/repair (nonthermal)	Acute inflammation (thermal)	Microstreaming (nonthermal)
Fracture (nonthermal)	Infection (thermal; local)	Acoustic streaming (nonthermal)
Pain (thermal or nonthermal)	Active epiphysis	Increased osteoblast and fibroblast proliferation (thermal and nonthermal)
Scar tissue (thermal or nonthermal depending on goals and acuteness)	Impaired sensation/cognition	Protein synthesis (nonthermal)
Calcium deposits	Pacemaker (local)	Increased cell and skin membrane permeability (nonthermal)
	Breast implants	
	Over central nervous system tissue	

Ultrasound intensity is the rate at which energy is being delivered per unit area. Ultrasound units generally offer intensities between 0.5 and 3.0 watts/square centimeter (W/cm^2). Spatial average intensity is the average intensity of the ultrasound output over the ultrasound transducer. The spatial average temporal average is the average amount of output over the on and off time, and the spatial average temporal peak is the average intensity of output during only the on time. The spatial average temporal peak is the measurement of the amount of energy being delivered to the tissue, which is often how intensities are expressed on ultrasound units. Intensity is decided based on how quickly one might want to heat the tissues (if performing a thermal intervention) as well as the patient's comfort level. Treatments that occur over bony areas require lower intensities because the ultrasound is being reflected. Students often find it frustrating that there are not specific intensity recommendations for certain diagnoses. The answer "it depends" is not a satisfying one, although it is true enough. There are some sources that suggest certain intensity ranges based on the acuteness of the injury, such as 0.1 to 0.3 W/cm^2 for acute injuries, 0.2 to 0.5 W/cm^2 for subacute injuries, and 0.3 to 0.8 W/cm^2 for chronic injuries.[7] There are also other recommendations based on the depth of the tissue being targeted, but none of these are firm dosages.

The final of the 4 main parameters set for ultrasound is time. The amount of time depends on several variables. The larger the size of the area being treated, the longer the treatment will be. Some sources say that one should apply ultrasound 1 minute/ultrasound head area.[7] This calculation would be 1 minute × the number of times the sound head fits over the lesion × the duty cycle in ratio form (1:4 for 20%, 1:1 for 50%, 1:0 for 100%).[7] This would then be influenced by the ultrasound head size. In addition, the reason for treating may affect the time; bone fracture healing will take longer, up to 20 minutes.[1] Keep in mind that when billing for ultrasound treatments, the set-up and follow-up to the treatment counts as billable time as much as the intervention itself. That means one may have applied a 5-minute ultrasound treatment to the patient, but it took 2 minutes to prepare the patient (eg, position correctly, drape, discuss contraindications) and another 1.5 minutes

	Table 5-2
	Procedures for Applying Therapeutic Ultrasound
Equipment Needed	• Ultrasound unit • Coupling medium • Alcohol wipes or antimicrobial agent • Towels
Treatment/ Parameters	• Confirm patient does not have contraindications. • Remove jewelry, clothing, etc from treatment area and inspect the skin. • Position patient for comfort and access to treatment area; drape for modesty/ warmth/clothing protection. • Have towels ready to wipe up the coupling medium once modality is complete. • Select appropriate sound head size. • Set parameters on ultrasound unit according to the goal of treatment: 1 or 3 MHz for depth, duty cycle based on thermal or nonthermal effects, and duration. • Apply coupling medium to area. • Apply ultrasound for duration required; maintain contact with the skin at all times and move sound head slowly but consistently (~ 4 cm/s). • Adjust intensity according to patient response and heat. • Check patient's response verbally during treatment and check the skin after treatment session. • Clean up after treatment; be sure to clean ultrasound head with alcohol wipe or other agent to prevent infection transmission.
Safety Considerations	• Move sound head slowly but consistently. • Keep sound head in contact with tissue. • Ensure you are using enough coupling medium. • Adjust intensity per patient response/comfort. • Ultrasound will feel more intense and possibly painful over bony areas.
Advantages	• Can address both chronic and acute injuries • Easy to use • Can penetrate to deeper tissues vs other modalities
Disadvantages	• Time consuming for larger areas • Clinician must be present for entire treatment

to clean up after and check the patient's skin. The actual duration of ultrasound, however, is different from billable time. Table 5-2 lists the parameter options for therapeutic ultrasound. Figures 5-9 and 5-10 show sample set-up screens for ultrasound.

There are various ways to apply ultrasound. Regardless of the parameter settings, a coupling medium is always needed. Generally, the coupling medium is ultrasound gel or lotion. However, one can also immerse the ultrasound head in water, use gel pads, or in the case of phonophoresis, apply various topical analgesics or creams to serve as a couplant for ultrasound, which will be discussed shortly. Figure 5-11 shows examples of coupling mediums.

Because of the potential to generate heat in the tissues, the sound head should be moved around the tissue to avoid the development of hot spots, which are painful. Clinicians should then make sure to move the sound head throughout the treatment session, with the aim to produce slow movements over the entire area. Ultrasound transducer head movement speed suggestions vary, but the general recommendation is to move the sound head approximately 4 cm/ second.[8] It does not matter if the sound head is moved in circles, lines, or other patterns, but the speed should be consistent and slow enough to provide uniform heating across the tissues.

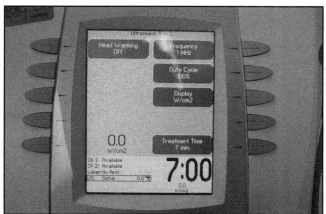

Figure 5-9. Sample set-up screen for ultrasound.

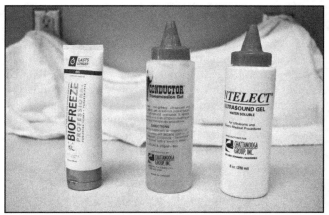

Figure 5-11. Coupling medium options (gel, lotion, Biofreeze).

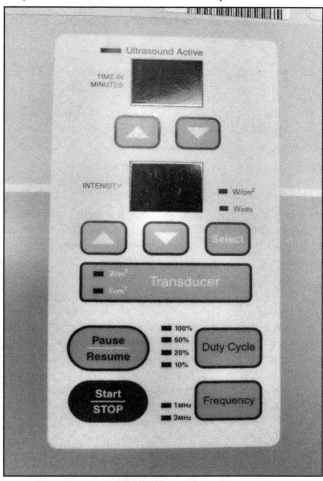

Figure 5-10. Sample set-up screen for ultrasound.

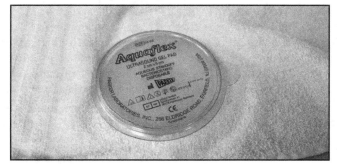

Figure 5-12. Gel bladder.

Also be aware of the type of tissue being treated and how it might absorb or reflect the ultrasound energy. As mentioned previously, tissues with a high collagen content absorb more ultrasound and heat faster than other tissues. Bony areas receiving ultrasound especially absorb heat quickly, and ultrasound can become uncomfortable as the periosteum heats. One should lower intensity when applying ultrasound over bony areas and be aware that certain tissues, such as blood, fat, and nerves, do not heat up as quickly with ultrasound.

One can also administer ultrasound in water. If coupling medium is not available or if the treatment area is small or irregularly shaped, or if the patient cannot tolerate the pressure of direct contact with the ultrasound head, you could attempt water immersion. Fill a plastic or rubber basin with water and submerge the body part receiving the treatment. Hold the ultrasound head 0.5 to 3.0 cm away from the treatment area and move the head parallel to the treatment area.

Another indirect coupling method may use a gel-filled bladder or gel pad (Figure 5-12).

ULTRASOUND IN COMBINATION WITH OTHER MODALITIES

Certain modalities can be and often are used in combination in the clinic. One study determined that applying a moist hot pack for 15 minutes before an ultrasound treatment yielded improved overall heating of the tissues, although it varied in terms of depth of penetration.[9]

Therapeutic Ultrasound

A later chapter will discuss using therapeutic ultrasound in combination with electrical stimulation. This combination yields the positive effects of both ultrasound and electrical stimulation.

Phonophoresis

Phonophoresis is the technique by which topical medications are administered via the use of ultrasound energy via intact skin. This is beneficial because the medications do not have to be administered orally or intravenously and the patient does not have to cope with systemic side effects of oral or intravenous medications. Phonophoresis is typically safe, painless, and easy to perform, and it is ideal for diagnoses such as strains, sprains, tendonitis, or bursitis.

Phonophoresis is thought to work via the increased tissue permeability created by the ultrasound treatment, both via the thermal and nonthermal effects. The ultrasound can increase cell permeability, and the vasodilation generated by thermal ultrasound settings might promote better diffusion of a drug.[10] The medication can then pass through the tissue into the area being treated.

Various medications are used with phonophoresis, the most common being anti-inflammatories such as hydrocortisone and dexamethasone, or analgesics such as lidocaine. These medications can be applied topically, allowed to dry, and then ultrasound gel applied to administer the treatment, or some medications can be embedded in a coupling medium. One study found that applying the medication and then placing an occlusive dressing of Tegaderm (3M) over the area yielded improved absorption of the medication.[11]

Phonophoresis parameters would be set based on similar goals as ultrasound; frequency will determine the depth of penetration; duty cycle will determine if the treatment generates thermal or nonthermal effects; intensity might be based on patient feedback or comfort; and time is relevant to the size of the area being treated and the goals of the treatment. If one is treating a patient for an inflammatory condition, avoid the thermal setting to prevent exacerbating the condition. Be attentive to patient response and check the patient's skin after the treatment. If the patient is already taking a drug orally, avoid administering it also with phonophoresis. Contraindications for phonophoresis are the same as for ultrasound. Table 5-3 provides the parameters for phonophoresis. See Box 5-2 for a phonophoresis-related research topic.

SAFETY CONCERNS

The primary concern for patients receiving therapeutic ultrasound or phonophoresis is the risk of burns or periosteal pain. As already mentioned, the application of ultrasound over bony areas will heat up the periosteum and cause pain. It has also been mentioned that the ultrasound head should be constantly moving to avoid creating a hot spot and burning the patient. Be sure to ask the patient for feedback and make parameter or application technique changes as needed.

Know all the contraindications and precautions for ultrasound application in order to avoid compromising a patient's safety. In addition to setting the parameters correctly and being attentive to the patient's response, know that ultrasound machines need to be regularly calibrated to ensure the machine is working correctly. If it is not, the patient may be unintentionally burned by the unit.

Be attentive to patient position, draping, as well as one's own body mechanics. Make sure to position the patient to access the area being treated, drape to provide warmth, modesty, as well as to protect clothing while you access the area, and raise or lower the patient as able to provide the treatment while adhering to proper body mechanics.

DOCUMENTATION

Two examples are provided to represent ultrasound and phonophoresis documentation.

Diagnosis: Patient with chronic stage IV pressure injury to the right calcaneus.

O: Applied pulsed ultrasound at 20% duty cycle, 3 MHz, 0.5 W/cm^2, × 5 minutes with 5-cm sound head to patient's right calcaneus to promote healing. Patient in supine with area draped and right lower extremity elevated to gain access to the area. Wound measured 2 × 2.8 × 0.8 cm before treatment. Patient had no complaints during or after the treatment.

Diagnosis: Patient with acute left knee bursitis with 8/10 pain.

O: Applied phonophoresis with 0.33% dexamethasone cream and use of Tegaderm dressing over left knee where patient reported 8/10 bursitis pain. Duty cycle 20%, frequency 3 MHz, 0.2 W/cm^2 × 5 minutes with 5-cm sound head to reduce pain and inflammation. Patient in short seated position with area draped. Patient reported no discomfort during the session and reported pain 6/10 after treatment.

	Table 5-3 Procedures for Applying Phonophoresis	
Equipment Needed	• Ultrasound unit • Coupling medium • Medication • Towels • Alcohol wipe or antimicrobial agent
Treatment/ Parameters	• Confirm patient does not have contraindications. • Remove jewelry, clothing, etc from treatment area and inspect the skin. • Position patient for comfort and access to treatment area; drape for modesty/ warmth/clothing protection. • Have towels ready to wipe up the coupling medium once modality is complete. • Select appropriate sound head size. • Set parameters on ultrasound unit according to goal of treatment: 1 or 3 MHz for depth, duty cycle based on thermal or nonthermal effects, and duration. • Apply medication to area if applying separately from the coupling medium; let dry and possibly apply occlusive dressing to enhance absorption. • Apply coupling medium to area if doing this separately from the medication. • Apply ultrasound for duration required; maintain contact with skin at all times and move sound head slowly but consistently. • Adjust intensity according to patient response and heat. • Check patient's response verbally during treatment and check the skin after treatment session. • Clean up after treatment; be sure to clean ultrasound head with an alcohol wipe or other agent to prevent infection transmission.
Safety Considerations	• Move sound head slowly but consistently. • Keep sound head in contact with tissue. • Adjust intensity per patient response/comfort. • Ultrasound will feel more intense and possibly painful over bony areas. • Do not apply phonophoresis of a medication the patient is already taking orally or intravenously.
Advantages	• Avoids negative side effects of oral/intravenous medications • Is safer than alternative medication treatments
Disadvantages	• Time consuming for larger areas • Clinician must be present for entire treatment • Absorption is variable depending on drug, tissue being treated, parameters of machine, etc

CONCLUSION

Ultrasound, like other therapeutic modalities, has been shown to be very beneficial for certain diagnosis and needs. It is limited to smaller treatment areas, but it can penetrate deeper than most other modalities. The parameters allow the therapist to specify the treatment for the patient's needs, and because it is typically a brief treatment, it can be easily incorporated into a patient's treatment plan. While there are some contraindications and precautions, and there is always the possibility of burning a patient if not performed correctly, patients often report they enjoy ultrasound treatment and it couples well with certain other modalities and interventions.

REVIEW QUESTIONS

1. What are the physiological effects of thermal ultrasound? Nonthermal?
2. List the contraindications for therapeutic ultrasound.
3. Discuss the 4 main parameters you need to set when applying an ultrasound treatment. What are they, and how do you determine how to set them?
4. How does phonophoresis work and what are its benefits?
5. You have a patient with an acute soft-tissue sprain after sliding into home base during a softball game last night. Pain is 7/10 with swelling noted in the area. What ultrasound parameters would you choose?
6. Your patient has a chronic venous stasis ulcer (1.2 × 1.4 × 0.02 cm) to the right lower extremity. What parameters for ultrasound would you select for this patient?
7. Document your treatment of the aforementioned 2 patients.
8. Discuss what safety concerns (aside from contraindications) you should be aware of or perform during an ultrasound treatment to maintain patient safety and comfort.

CASE STUDY 1

Your patient is a 17-year-old woman who tore her right anterior cruciate ligament during a soccer match 6 weeks ago. She underwent surgical repair and has been coming to outpatient rehabilitation for therapy. She has limited knee extension with passive range of motion of 8 to 101 degrees and continued pain of 3/10 at rest and 6/10 with therapy or vigorous activity. She also still shows some swelling in the area, especially at the end of the day.
1. What tissues were injured?
2. What are the physiological effects of this intervention?
3. What contraindications should you be mindful of when considering ultrasound for this patient?
4. What parameters would you suggest for this patient? Why? How would they change based on the goal of the intervention?
5. If the patient is showing no improvement in her pain after 1 week of ultrasound, what alterations to the therapy intervention could be made to achieve improved results?

CASE STUDY 2

Your patient was in a car accident 8 weeks ago and suffered significant injury to her left hip and proximal femur, requiring her to be in a cast for the duration of her healing process. Her surgery required the insertion of several pins and screws. Now she comes to therapy for gait training, transfer training, and deconditioning. The physical therapist evaluation shows the patient has limited hip extension due to being casted for 8 weeks and, thus, gait is affected on the left side, causing a shortened step length on the right. The patient has some pain, 3 to 4/10, with hip extension. She reports fatigue with prolonged gait attempts and is unable to walk more than 100 feet (30.5 cm) without requiring a rest break.
1. What ultrasound parameters would you suggest for the patient's need for soft-tissue shortening?
2. What effect do the patient's pins and screws have on the ultrasound treatment?
3. What contraindications should you consider when applying ultrasound to this patient?
4. What other interventions (not necessarily ultrasound) would you recommend for this patient? Why?

REFERENCES

1. Della Rocca GJ. The science of ultrasound therapy for fracture healing. *Indian J Orthop.* 2009;43(2):121-126.
2. Mongan E. Ultrasound accelerating wound healing. *McKnight's Long-Term Care News.* 2015;36(9):8.
3. Liao JC, Chen WJ, Chen LH, Lai PL, Keorochana G. Low-intensity pulsed ultrasound enhances healing of laminectomy chip bone grafts on spinal fusion: a model of posterolateral intertransverse fusion in rabbits. *J Trauma.* 2011;70(4):863-869.
4. Lovric V, Ledger M, Goldberg J, et al. The effects of low-intensity pulsed ultrasound on tendon-bone healing in a transosseous-equivalent sheep rotator cuff model. *Knee Surg Sports Traumatol Arthrosc.* 2012;21(2):466-475.
5. Kocaoğlu B, Cabukoglu C, Ozeras N, Seyhan M, Karahan M, Yalcin S. The effect of therapeutic ultrasound on metallic implants: a study in rats. *Arch Phys Med Rehabil.* 2011;92(11):1858-1862.
6. Draper DO, Castel JC, Castel D. Rate of temperature increase in human muscle during 1 MHz and 3 MHz continuous ultrasound. *J Orthop Sports Phys Ther.* 1995;22(4):142-150.
7. Electrotherapy on the Web. Ultrasound dose calculation. 2020. Accessed January 23, 2020. http://www.electrotherapy.org/modality/ultrasound-dose-calculation#Compiling%20the%20treatment%20dose
8. Weaver SL, Demchak TJ, Stone MB, Brucker JB, Burr PO. Effect of transducer velocity on intramuscular temperature during a 1-MHz ultrasound treatment. *J Orthop Sports Phys Ther.* 2006;36(5):320-325.
9. Draper DO, Harris ST, Schulthies S, Durrant E, Knight KL, Ricard M. Hot-Pack and 1-MHz ultrasound treatment have an additive effect on muscle temperature increase. *J Athl Train.* 1998;33(1):21-24.
10. Klaiman MD, Shrader JA, Danoff JV, Hicks JE, Pesce WJ, Ferland J. Phonophoresis versus ultrasound in the treatment of common musculoskeletal conditions. *Med Sci Sports Exerc.* 1998;30(9):1349-1355.
11. Saliba S, Dilaawar JM, Perrin DH, Gieck J, Weltman A. Phonophoresis and the absorption of dexamethasone in the presence of an occlusive dressing. *J Athl Train.* 2007;42(3):349-354.

Mechanical Agents

Chapter 6

Hydrotherapy

KEY TERMS Buoyancy | Debridement | Eschar | Exudate | Granulation tissue | Hydrostatic pressure | Maceration | Nosocomial | Purulent | Resistance | Thermal conductivity | Viscosity

KEY ABBREVIATIONS CHF | MS | PSI | VO$_2$

CHAPTER OBJECTIVES

1. Discuss the physical properties of water and how those apply to therapy interventions.
2. Describe the physiological effects of hydrotherapy.
3. Consider the ways hydrotherapy is applied to physical therapy interventions.
4. Categorize the indications and contraindications for hydrotherapy interventions.
5. Apply knowledge of hydrotherapy parameters to case scenarios.
6. Document hydrotherapy interventions correctly in a patient's chart.

INTRODUCTION

To understand how hydrotherapy can be used in therapeutic interventions, it is important first to understand the physical properties of water. These properties influence the physiological effects of water on the body and include thermal conductivity, buoyancy, hydrostatic pressure, and resistance. This section will first address each of these properties to better understand how water affects the body.

Water can transmit heat (or cold) via conduction and convection. That is, if someone sticks their hand in warm water and holds it, the heat is transmitted via conduction. If the water swirls around one's hand, heat is being transmitted via convection. The movement of the water transmits the heat (or cold) faster, making it a very effective method of heating or cooling a patient's tissues. This is the concept of thermal conductivity, and many therapists use water's ability to transmit heat or cold to patients to meet therapeutic goals.

The fact that a person will float in a pool is a demonstration of buoyancy. The amount of fluid dispersed by the body affects the upward thrust of the body. This is because the density of the human body is less than the density of water. Swimming in the ocean causes one to float more easily than in a pool; the addition of salt affects the density of the water and the body will float higher. The same principle applies when wearing flotation devices. Figures 6-1 and 6-2 show different types of pool equipment for flotation or resistance training. Owing to the concept of buoyancy, a patient may have an easier time performing exercises when immersed in a pool vs on dry land. Flotation devices can further assist with weightbearing restrictions or pain. Figure 6-3 shows a person using a pool noodle for flotation, and Figure 6-4 shows different types of flotation devices in the water.

Hydrostatic pressure refers to the pressure of fluid exerted on a body immersed in that fluid. Hydrostatic pressure increases with depth, so if one were to stand in a pool up to the neck, there would be more pressure on the distal

Memolo J.
Therapeutic Agents for the Physical Therapist Assistant
(pp 59-71). © 2022 SLACK Incorporated.

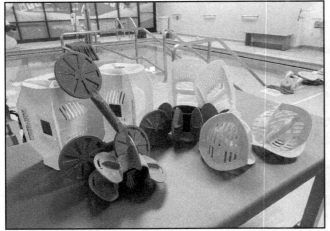

Figure 6-1. Pool equipment.

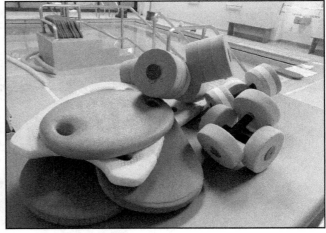

Figure 6-2. Pool equipment.

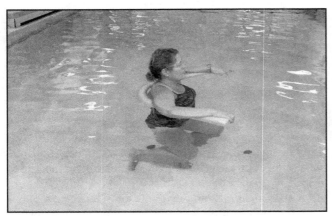

Figure 6-3. Patient using pool noodle for floating.

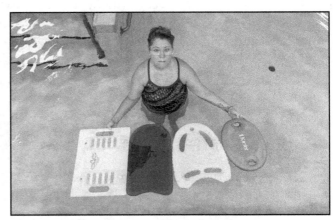

Figure 6-4. Different flotation paddles in the pool.

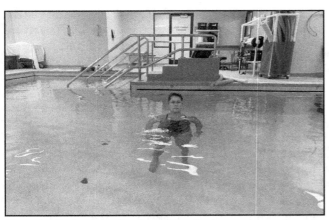

Figure 6-5. Patient in pool up to shoulders/neck.

lower extremities than the upper body (Figure 6-5). This pressure would be less if one were in water only up to the hips (Figure 6-6). Think about a deep-sea diver. A human body can dive only so deep because the hydrostatic pressure increases the deeper the diver goes. Go too deep and the weight of the water above and around the divers will crush them. Because of this pressure, vertical immersion in water can promote circulation and reduce edema, especially in lower extremities.

Finally, let's discuss resistance. Walking through water that is only 3 inches deep is not very difficult. Now think about walking through water that is up to the knees. Now up to the midchest. It becomes progressively more difficult. This is resistance. Water viscosity, or thickness, provides this resistance and it increases with the amount of the body immersed and the speed of motion. In an aquatic setting, a patient can wear fins or paddles to additionally increase the resistance. Figure 6-7 shows the different resistance options in paddles depending on whether the flaps are open or closed; closed flaps result in more resistance. Figure 6-8 shows a person wearing a lower extremity fin to increase resistance. This resistance can be used by a therapist to assist in strengthening as well as endurance training, while the patient remains safe from falls.

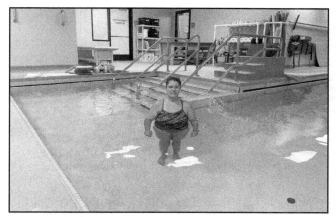

Figure 6-6. Patient in pool up to hips.

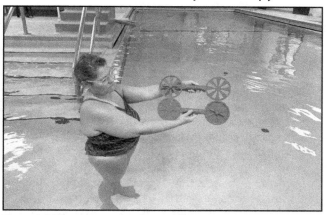

Figure 6-7. Flaps open vs closed on paddles.

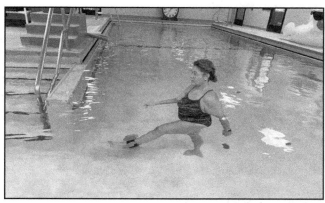

Figure 6-8. Patient wearing lower extremity fin to increase resistance.

PHYSIOLOGICAL EFFECTS OF HYDROTHERAPY

The effects of water on the body are many, and they include cleansing, musculoskeletal, cardiovascular, respiratory, renal, psychological, and thermal effects. This section will discuss each one in detail.

Cleansing Effects

The use of water as a cleanser is one most are familiar with; what may be less familiar is that the use of water, especially agitated water, can loosen debris in a wound and can soften tissue that might otherwise be difficult to debride. Necrotic tissue, or tough, dead tissue called *eschar*, can prove difficult to remove with traditional wound-care tools. A patient once suffered a seizure and then turned over his kerosene-fueled heating element at his house. The hot kerosene poured over his arm, causing third-degree burns. In the wound care clinic, the physical therapist assistant's job was to remove the dead, black tissue to promote proper healing, but it was difficult to do with scissors and a scalpel because the tissue was tough and leathery. The therapist used a hydrotherapy tank and immersed the patient's arm for a period, which allowed that hard tissue to soften so it could be more easily cut away.

Wounds can also have exudate, sometimes bloody or purulent. A hydrotherapy treatment can clean the exudate out of the wound to keep the wound clean and prevent or decrease infection. Antimicrobials can also be added to the water to further help with the healing process.

Musculoskeletal Effects

A previous section already discussed water's buoyancy and resistance properties. These properties have a direct effect on a patient's musculoskeletal system. Buoyancy allows for decreased weightbearing, which is great for patients who have weightbearing restrictions, such as after a surgery, or for patients who have pain with weightbearing,

such as after an injury, when pregnant, or with a joint-integrity issue like arthritis. Buoyancy can also help patients feel safer; they are not going to fall on a hard surface and injure themselves.

Resistance also promotes improvement in the musculoskeletal system. Resistance allows for strengthening and can be adjusted by the speed of movement as well as the depth of immersion. Patients who have neuromuscular diseases, such as Parkinson disease, a cerebrovascular accident (CVA), or multiple sclerosis (MS) can benefit from the resistance water provides during therapy sessions. The use of resistance also can promote improvements in balance, again without the fear of a patient falling and hurting themself.[1]

Cardiovascular Effects

Hydrostatic pressure is the primary property that affects cardiovascular function during hydrotherapy interventions. This chapter previously discussed that the deeper the immersion, the more pressure the water exerts on the body. Thus, if a person is standing vertically in the water, the lower extremities receive more pressure than the upper body. This acts as a form of compression, moving blood and other fluid up toward the heart.[2]

In addition, water's effects on the heart's function include improved aerobic capacity,[3,4] reduction of heart rate (HR), and an increase in stroke volume.[2] A patient's maximal oxygen consumption (VO_2) also has been shown to decrease with hydrotherapy exercise,[4] and a patient's HR and systolic blood pressure response to exercises is reduced with hydrotherapy programs.[5]

Remember that water temperature can affect cardiovascular function. Warm water promotes vasodilation and increased blood flow, whereas cold water vasoconstricts. A systematic review of studies investigating the use of hydrotherapy showed that warm water immersion not only caused vasodilation and increased blood flow, but it also reduced arterial stiffness, improved oxygenation, and yielded effects similar to those of physical activity.[6]

Respiratory Effects

Like the cardiovascular system, the respiratory system is affected primarily by hydrostatic pressure in water. As water exerts its pressure on the body, so too are the lungs compressed. This can increase the work of breathing when submerged in water, and the deeper the submersion, the harder the work.[7] While hydrostatic pressure's effects on vital capacity for uninjured individuals seems limited, it has been shown to improve vital capacity in patients with spinal cord injuries.[8,9] It has also been shown to be less likely to cause exercise-induced asthma.[10,11]

Renal Effects

Again, hydrostatic pressure plays a role in the effects of water on renal function. Think about the last time you went swimming. After being in the water for a while, one may feel the need to urinate. Research has shown that immersion in water can lower plasma renin activity and decrease renal vascular pressure.[12] Immersion in water causes a decrease in aldosterone and antidiuretic hormone, the hormone that prevent diuresis, which yields sodium and potassium excretion and results in the need to use the bathroom.[12,13]

Psychological Effects

Unless one is afraid of water, one may recognize that being in water can provide certain psychological benefits. Warm water can be relaxing or soothing, while cool water can be invigorating. Some studies have been conducted to determine the psychological benefits of water therapy; a 2014 study of a patient with mild dementia determined that an aquatic exercise program can improve psychological well-being per results on a memory and well-being scale.[14] Another study looking at older patients with depression showed a decrease in anxiety and depression after 12 weeks of aquatic exercise.[15] Because being in the water can reduce pain during therapy interventions, a patient may be more relaxed and willing to participate.

Thermal Effects

This section will discuss the effects water can have on the body with respect to its temperature. Thermotherapy induces vasodilation, increased blood flow, pain reduction due to the Gate Control theory, healing, and increased flexibility. Cryotherapy causes vasoconstriction, pain reduction, slowed nerve conduction velocity, and anesthesia. These effects can occur simultaneously with the previously listed effects specific to water therapy, and they influence the indications for water-based therapy interventions.

INDICATIONS AND CONTRAINDICATIONS OF HYDROTHERAPY

Now that the physiological effects of hydrotherapy have been discussed, this section can dive into the reasons why one uses hydrotherapy and why one would not.

Indications for hydrotherapy are plenty, and many of them have already been discussed. As mentioned in the Thermotherapy and Cryotherapy chapters (Chapters 3 and 4, respectively), water can provide heating or cooling effects. Thusly, any indication for hot or cold therapy would also be an indication for hydrotherapy. To promote circulation, control pain, or increase soft-tissue extensibility, one would choose to use warm water. To create an analgesic and possibly anesthetic effect, address acute soft-tissue injuries, or reduce swelling, one might choose cool water. Water is beneficial in that it can cover large areas of the skin and contour to those areas well, unlike a moist hot pack or a cold pack. However, the penetration of heat or cold is superficial.

Another indication for hydrotherapy would be any diagnosis or need for water exercise. Again, some of these have already been mentioned. If patients cannot perform land-based exercises because of obesity, pain, joint instability, bone density loss, or weightbearing restrictions, water exercises would be indicated. Patients with neurological impairments such as CVA, spinal cord injury, MS, or Parkinson disease could benefit from the proprioceptive input water provides, as well as its assurance of safety from falls. Patients with poor cardiovascular tolerance of land-based exercises might perform better in the water. Patients who are pregnant may find water exercises to be more comfortable because of the decreased weightbearing and the lesser effects on the heart, not to mention positive benefits to lower-extremity swelling. Patients with exercise-induced asthma may also prefer water-based exercises to land-based. As long as these patients do not have contraindications, which will be addressed shortly, hydrotherapy could be beneficial. Box 6-1 offers a research topic on the use of aquatic therapy on patients with Parkinson disease.

Water can additionally provide a reduction of pain. The warmth or coolness of the water contributes to this via the Gate Control theory or slowed nerve conduction velocity, as does the decreased weightbearing generated by buoyancy. Patients with pain for any reason may then find water therapy to be preferable.

Owing to the effects of hydrostatic pressure, as well as the possible contributions of cold water, edema reduction is another indication for hydrotherapy. However, one would want to avoid using warm water with patients who have edema or are prone to edema.

Wound care is a significant indication for hydrotherapy. There are options to use large tanks to provide agitation for cleansing and softening of tissue; the use of pulsed lavage devices can also clean and debride a wound without the need for immersion. The use of whirlpool tanks to clean wounds can run the risk of a nosocomial infection if the tanks are not cleaned properly, so the therapist must be sure the tank is clean before use. Interestingly, the American Physical Therapy Association states in its Choosing Wisely campaign that one should not use a whirlpool for wound management for this very reason: Whirlpools cause the risk of cross-contamination and the agitation can damage delicate tissues.[16] Many clinics are moving away from having large whirlpool tanks because they can be time consuming to fill, empty, and clean, as well as pricey. Instead, many wound care clinicians prefer the use of wound irrigation or pulsed lavage systems. Box 6-2 offers a research topic on the subject of using hydrotherapy and ultrasound for wound care.

Although hydrotherapy has many possible indications, one should be aware of all the contraindications. These contraindications can be divided into those that apply for local immersion, total immersion, or nonimmersion hydrotherapy interventions, although one will find that many overlap.

Local immersion hydrotherapy should be avoided for patients with maceration in the area to be treated. If maceration is already present, the tissue is compromised and a wound could form or, if a wound is already present, it could grow larger. A recent skin graft or any unstable tissue would not be appropriate for hydrotherapy until more healing has occurred. In addition, if the patient is bleeding in the area to be immersed, one would avoid that. Exposure to water will only exacerbate the bleeding, and the risk of contamination is also very high. Similarly, one should avoid local immersion if the patient has an active infection in the area to be immersed. This is because one neither wants to exacerbate or spread the infection (because warm temperatures

promote circulation), and one would not want to spread the infection to other patients. It may sound strange because wound care is an indication for hydrotherapy; however, if a patient has a wound and a therapist is considering aquatic interventions that are not wound-care based, the therapist may want to avoid it at the risk of causing an infection.

As with any modality that could have a thermal effect, ensure that the patient has intact sensation to avoid the risk of accidentally burning the patient. If the patient has impaired cognition this, too, could yield inaccurate feedback from the patient.

Total immersion comes with its own set of contraindications, although some, such as bleeding or infections, carry over from local immersion.[17] Although pregnancy is an indication for hydrotherapy, it is contraindicated if the water is too warm. Too-warm water, especially in the first trimester, can be damaging to a fetus, so excessively warm water should be avoided. Similarly, patients with MS can benefit from hydrotherapy, but the water cannot be too warm. Patients with MS demonstrate an exacerbation of their symptoms when subjected to excessive heat, so it is important to check the water temperature to avoid causing an exacerbation.

Other contraindications for total immersion include cardiac instability, such as uncontrolled hypertension or chronic/congestive heart failure (CHF). Water can affect cardiac output, and the pressure exerted can increase circulation to the heart. Patients with CHF already have hearts that cannot adequately handle the load placed on them, so avoid adding to that load. Some studies have found that patients with CHF can benefit from certain types of aquatic exercises, but it is wise to be at least cautious with this population.

In addition, patients with severe/uncontrolled epilepsy or suicidal patients are contraindicated for total immersion therapy.[17] Make sure the patients are safe; a patient having a seizure in the pool would not be safe. Patients who are suicidal could be at risk for injury or worse if placed in a total immersion scenario. Bowel incontinence is a hard contraindication, whereas urinary incontinence is considered a precaution by some; it depends on the patient and the situation. A fear of water is also considered at least a precaution, but

Table 6-1

Indications, Contraindications, and Physiological Effects of Hydrotherapy

Indications	Contraindications	Physiological Effects
Wound care	Maceration	Remove debris
Edema reduction	Active infection	Use antimicrobials to promote cleansing
Musculoskeletal problems	Hemorrhage	Decrease weightbearing
Neurological diagnoses	Impaired sensation/cognition	Strengthening
Decreased cardiac endurance	Water temperature too warm (MS, pregnancy)	Increase venous circulation
Pregnancy	Cardiac instability	Increase cardiac volume and output
Exercise-induced asthma	Suicidal patients	Decreased HR, systolic blood pressure, and VO_2 response to exercise
Pain	Severe epilepsy	Increased work of breathing
Edema	Incontinence	Decreased exercise-induced asthma
Wounds/burns	Fear of the water (precaution)	Diuresis
Diagnoses that prohibit land-based activity	Peripheral vascular disease	Relaxing or invigorating, depending on temperature

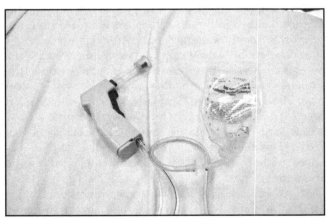

Figure 6-9. Pulsed lavage system.

the patient would have to be comfortable with the therapy interventions to make participation useful.[16]

Nonimmersion therapy contraindications still include those such as infections or bleeding, as well as maceration around a wound bed. Generally, one should be sure that pulsed lavage or similar nonimmersion hydrotherapies are required and useful. That is, nonimmersion therapies are not effective if the goal is to achieve cardiovascular, respiratory, or musculoskeletal improvements. As mentioned previously, there are some recommendations that pulsed lavage be used instead of a whirlpool because of cross-contamination and intensity of agitation to the wound. Table 6-1 lists the indications, contraindications, and physiological effects of hydrotherapy.

APPLICATION METHODS

Pulsed Lavage or Nonimmersion Therapy

Nonimmersion irrigation, often referred to as *pulsed lavage*, refers to the use of a device that performs hydrotherapy to a localized area without the need for immersion. This is beneficial for patients with contraindications to immersion (either localized or total) and avoids the concerns listed earlier regarding cross-contamination in wounds. Pulsed lavage systems are frequently used during wound care interventions because they can offer enough pressure (measured in pounds/square inch or psi) to cleanse and debride a wound without causing tissue damage. The pressure can be adjusted, and pressure for typical wound care interventions ranges from 4 to 12 psi,[18] although higher pressures can be used and have, in some cases, been shown to be beneficial.[19] This is in comparison with other irrigation methods, such as bulb syringes or the use of a whirlpool, which provide either too little or too much pressure. In addition, pulsed lavage systems are relatively inexpensive, portable, and easy to use, meaning they can be used in a variety of settings. Pulsed lavage systems (Figure 6-9) include a handpiece connected via a tube to an irrigation solution, most often sterile saline. Handpieces can have a variety of tips to better access the wound, including long, thin tips to access tunneling wounds. The handpiece is also then connected to some form of suction; as the trigger is pulled to release the water onto the wound, the suction draws the contaminated fluid back into a containment canister that can be disposed

Table 6-2

Procedures for Applying Nonimmersion Therapy (Pulsed Lavage)

Equipment Needed	• Nonimmersion device/pulsed lavage system and all accessories (eg, tips, tubing) • Irrigation fluid (usually sterile saline) • Towels
Treatment/ Parameters	• Confirm patient does not have contraindications. • Remove jewelry, clothing, etc from treatment area and inspect the skin. • Position patient for comfort and access to treatment area; drape for modesty/warmth/clothing protection. • Have towels ready to wipe up excess water once modality is complete. • Therapist should don proper gown, gloves, mask, and face shield for infection control. • Select appropriate tip. • Connect handpiece to sterile saline bag and collection unit. Saline should be warmed up before use. • Turn on unit and select pressure. Up to 15 psi is usually sufficient for debridement. • Perform treatment until area is hydrated/debrided sufficiently. • Can follow up with remaining wound care interventions as needed, including wound dressing. • Check patient's response verbally during treatment and check the skin after treatment session. • Clean up after treatment; wipe down handpiece if reusing with same patient, or dispose of all equipment. • Can be performed 1 time/day every day if needed.
Safety Considerations	• Monitor for patient pain. • If patient is bleeding during treatment, may need to stop treatment or decrease pressure.
Advantages	• Treatment is relatively inexpensive compared to whirlpool • Can be applied to localized area • Can reduce risk of infection/contamination • Appropriate for patients contraindicated for localized or total body immersion • Less time consuming
Disadvantages	• There is a cost for replacing tubing, tips, and handpieces with new patients/applications • Patient does not benefit from buoyancy, resistance, or hydrostatic pressure

of. The tubing, handpiece, and tips are also made to be disposable to avoid cross-contamination. Table 6-2 details the procedure for applying nonimmersion hydrotherapy.

Localized Immersion

Localized immersion of a patient's extremity is typically performed using a whirlpool. These come in a variety of sizes and heights, and these allow for patients to immerse the body part in question in the water without affecting the rest of the body. The whirlpool itself is often stainless steel with a motor connected to a turbine that is submerged in the water (Figure 6-10). The turbine/motor system can usually be rotated so the water agitation is somewhat adjustable and can be pointed at or away from the body part being submerged. It is recommended that the agitation be pointed toward wounds requiring cleansing or that have necrotic tissue or eschar, whereas fragile wounds or wounds with new healing would benefit from the agitation pointed away. A patient can receive wound care via a whirlpool set-up, although the risk for cross-contamination is high and, as previously stated, a nonimmersion method might be as beneficial if not more so. A patient can also perform localized exercises in a whirlpool, including range of motion exercises, and can benefit from the whirlpool for pain relief.

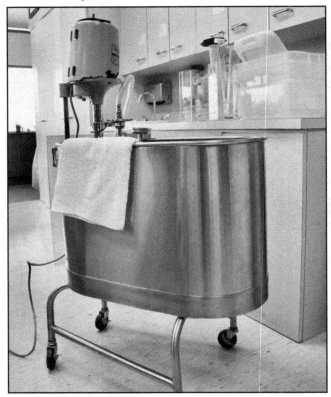

Figure 6-10. Whirlpool.

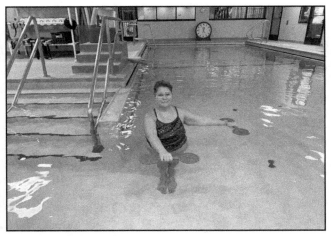

Figure 6-11. Patient using paddles.

The costs of filling, maintaining, and cleaning whirlpools, not to mention the challenges of transferring and positioning patients for whirlpool use, means that fewer therapy settings use these tools, but they are something you may encounter in your therapy settings. See Table 6-3 for the steps of applying localized immersion hydrotherapy.

There are no official temperature parameters for specific interventions; however, there are some agreed-on ranges of temperatures that constitute cold, warm, or hot water. Cold water can be defined as 32°F to 79°F, tepid is 79°F to 92°F, neutral warmth is 92°F to 96°F, mild warmth is 96°F to 98°F, hot is 99°F to 104°F, and very hot is 104°F to 110°F. Some sources indicate that you should not exceed 110°F because of the risk of burns as well as increased risk for elevated blood pressure and dizziness. For a point of comparison, the Centers for Disease Control and Prevention recommends that hot tub temperatures not exceed 104°F.[20] Temperature recommendations correlate to treatment goals. Cold water is appropriate for acute injuries or inflammation, swelling, or pain. Warm and hot temperatures help with tissue extensibility and pain control, including for chronic conditions. One might consider that temperatures between 79°F and 92°F is tepid or neutral warmth, which is what one might expect to see in a therapy pool. Table 6-4 includes the temperatures and therapeutic applications for each.

Full-Body Immersion

Full-body immersion usually takes place in a pool setting, although there are other options. A Hubbard tank, for example, is a large tank that allows full-body immersion. It was originally created for the treatment of polio, and soon thereafter it was used for wound care, primarily for the treatment of burns.[21] Hubbard tanks are rarely used because of the costs associated with using and maintaining them, and other methods of wound care are easier to use, cheaper to access, and come with less risk of infection. Hubbard tanks also require a great deal of space, which many clinics simply do not have. Still, there is a chance of seeing one in certain settings.

A therapy pool offers the opportunity for a patient to be fully immersed in water to perform exercises. Figures 6-11 through 6-14 show various ways patients can use equipment to exercise in the therapy pool. In this way, the patient can benefit from the physical properties of hydrostatic pressure, resistance, and buoyancy, as well as the thermal effects water can provide. The Mayo Clinic states that temperatures between 28.3°C and 31.1°C (83°F to 88°F) is comfortable for water exercise.[22] Recreational pools, by contrast, range between 78°F and 82°F.[23] There are a few exceptions or considerations to this recommendation. As mentioned in the contraindications section, individuals who are pregnant and in their first trimester should avoid excessively warm/hot water. Patients with MS should also be mindful of water temperature; although pool exercise is great for this patient population, overheating can cause exacerbation of the disease. According to the National Multiple Sclerosis Society, temperatures between 80°F and 84°F is optimal.[24]

In a pool setting, patients can decide how immersed to be, and they can move freely in. Some clinic therapy pools are relatively small, and some have mechanical lifts to raise and lower patients in and out of the pool if they cannot walk in and out. A pool can offer the patient the opportunity to move without the fear of falling and can reduce

Table 6-3
Procedures for Applying Localized Immersion

Equipment Needed	• Access to warm/cold water • Whirlpool tank with turbine • Heated, well-ventilated space • (Heated) towels
Treatment/ Parameters	• Confirm patient does not have contraindications. • Remove jewelry, clothing, etc from treatment area and inspect the skin. • Have towels ready to wipe up excess water once modality is complete. • Fill tank with water of appropriate temperature. • Position patient for comfort/access; drape for modesty/warmth/clothing protection. Ensure there is no pressure on limb that is submerged. If patient has wound dressing, remove before treatment. No clothing should be in the tank because it can get tangled in the turbine. • If performing wound care, therapist should don gown, gloves, mask, and face shield. • Direct turbine to point at or away from treatment area. • Turn on unit; stay with patient during session and monitor response. • Can follow up with remaining wound care interventions as needed, including wound dressing. • Check patient's response verbally during treatment and check the skin after treatment. • Clean up after treatment; wipe down whirlpool according to directions provided. • Typically applied 10 to 30 min depending on treatment goal.
Safety Considerations	• Monitor for patient pain. • If patient is bleeding during treatment, will need to stop treatment. • Monitor patient vital signs and discontinue if they stray from normal. • Patient might be chilled or lightheaded after treatment.
Advantages	• Appropriate for both wound care and exercise interventions, as well as for heat/cold transfer • Patient can move extremity while submerged in water
Disadvantages	• Size of tank limits exercises that can be performed • Risk for cross-contamination • Time consuming to fill, empty, and clean • Costly to fill and heat water

Table 6-4
Water Temperatures and Therapeutic Applications

Temperature, °F	Therapeutic Applications
32 to 79	Cold: acute inflammation, swelling, pain
79 to 92	Tepid: exercise, wounds
92 to 96	Neutral warm: wound care and spasticity
96 to 98	Mild warmth: treatment of burns
98 to 104	Hot: pain management
104 to 110	Very hot: chronic osteoarthritis or rheumatoid arthritis, for ROM

Abbreviation: ROM, range of motion.

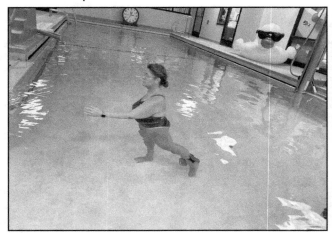

Figure 6-12. Patient using lower extremity fins.

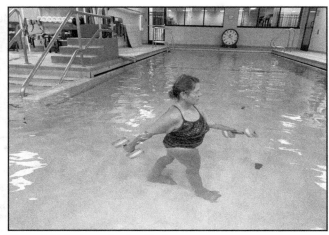

Figure 6-13. Patient using dumbbells.

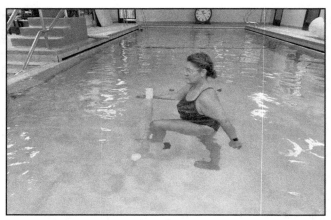

Figure 6-14. Patient using pool noodle.

weightbearing and pain. Exercise in a pool can be closed-chain or open-chain depending on positioning and the use of flotation devices. The patient should not have any of the contraindications listed previously to qualify for full-body immersion, and the patient should be careful entering and exiting the pool to avoid slipping. Table 6-5 lists the steps for applying full-body immersion hydrotherapy.

SAFETY CONCERNS

Safety considerations for hydrotherapy of course correlate to any possible precautions or contraindications. However, there are a few other red flags to watch for when working with your patient. For example, we discussed the effects of water on the cardiovascular system. Because HR responds differently to exercise in the water, monitoring HR as a means to assess the patient's response may be unreliable. Instead, one may want to use a Borg Rating of Perceived Exertion Scale, which offers a scale of how hard the patient perceives they are working. The scale ranges from 6, which is no exertion at all, to 20, which is maximal exertion. Patients can rate how hard the exercise is, and

a 12 to 14 on the scale correlates to a moderate-intensity exercise.[25] If the patient rates the activity as a 19 when the goal was a 13, one would have the patient slow down or take a break to decrease the perceived intensity.

Because hydrotherapy can cause increased work of breathing, it is important to monitor patients for respiratory distress. There are tools, such as the Modified Borg Dyspnea Scale or the Modified Medical Research Council Dyspnea Scale, that assess a patient's shortness of breath. One can also monitor the patient's respiratory rate and oxygen saturation. Patients with respiratory illnesses should especially be monitored during water therapy interventions.

Another respiratory concern is for patients with asthma. Hydrotherapy can be beneficial for patients who have exercise-induced asthma. However, the chemicals used to clean the pools can exacerbate asthma symptoms, so it is important to monitor patients with asthma carefully during the treatment session.

When performing wound care, one will want to view the wound bed and surrounding tissue to make sure further damage is not occurring. Owing to the increased risk of contamination and infection, check the wound every session to ensure there are no signs or symptoms of new infection.

Hydrostatic pressure can help relieve edema in the extremities submerged in water; however, warm water can counter those effects. If a therapist is treating a patient with edema or with the hopes of addressing that problem, or if the patient is prone to edema, the therapist may want to consider the water temperature and how it could negatively affect the severity of edema.

Water temperature can negatively affect a patient's body in other ways, also. Too cold and the patient may suffer from hypothermia; too warm and the patient could have hyperthermia. Too-cold water can negatively affect heart function, reflexes, and blood pressure. Too-hot water can result in higher blood pressure, dizziness, or burns.

	Table 6-5 **Procedures for Applying Full-Body Immersion**	
Equipment Needed	• Pool, with appropriate heating and ventilation • Space for patients to change/shower • Safety equipment, including nonslip area around pool • Infection control equipment • Towels • Thermometer
Treatment/ Parameters	• Confirm patient does not have contraindications. • Remove jewelry, clothing, etc from treatment area and inspect the skin. • Have towels ready for patient to dry off after therapy session. • Ensure pool is at proper temperature by checking thermometer. • Ensure all safety equipment is present and readily available. • Patient and therapist should wear swimming suits. • Assist patient (if necessary) into pool. • Perform activities planned. These could be endurance activities such as walking, resistance training, balance training, etc. • Use flotation devices to assist with buoyancy and/or resistance equipment for strengthening. • Monitor patient's response to all interventions, including vital signs and Borg scale. • Stay with patient the entire session. • At completion, assist patient out of the pool (if necessary) and wrap patient with towels to prevent chilling.
Safety Considerations	• Monitor patient's vitals and fatigue levels during session; stop session if patient strays from normal values. • Be ready to adjust or change interventions depending on patient response. • Stay with patient the entire session to prevent potential drowning or injury. • Make sure patient is safe getting into and out of pool and when going to locker room to change clothes. The patient may need assistance with this step.
Advantages	• Patient can move freely in pool • Patient can perform activities that meet cardiovascular, respiratory, strengthening, or endurance goals • Patient will reap benefits of buoyancy and hydrostatic pressure, including reduced pain and weight bearing
Disadvantages	• Patient is at higher risk of falling getting into and out of pool • Risk of cross-contamination in pool if other patients have infections or are incontinent • Risk of drowning

Drowning is always a concern when working with water. The therapist will stay close to the patient in the water and will know where and how to use the safety equipment in the pool area in case of an emergency. As mentioned in the contraindications section, avoid full-immersion therapy with patients who have high risk factors for drowning, such as uncontrolled epilepsy or suicidal thoughts. In many cases there are at least 2 therapists in the pool area at any given time to be prepared for emergency situations.

Finally, a general concern is that of pool maintenance and safety. Patients should know and understand the pool rules and follow them; an example is provided in Figure 6-15. Pools and whirlpools need to be cleaned regularly using the appropriate materials. Whirlpools need to be checked regularly to ensure the electrical components work correctly and will not cause electrical shock. Pools and whirlpool areas need to be well ventilated because of the use of chemical cleansers.

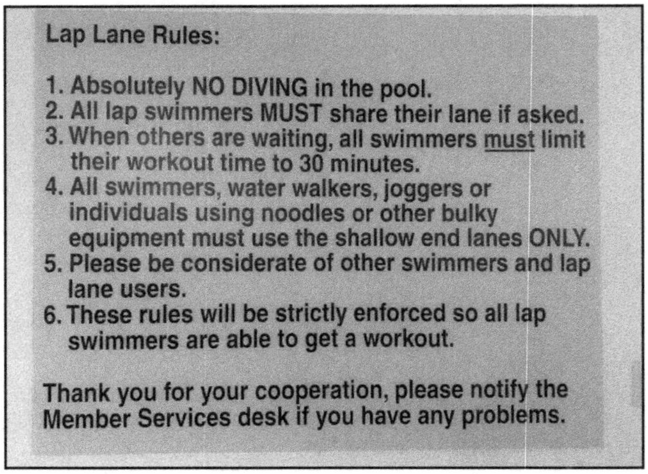

Lap Lane Rules:

1. Absolutely NO DIVING in the pool.
2. All lap swimmers MUST share their lane if asked.
3. When others are waiting, all swimmers <u>must</u> limit their workout time to 30 minutes.
4. All swimmers, water walkers, joggers or individuals using noodles or other bulky equipment must use the shallow end lanes ONLY.
5. Please be considerate of other swimmers and lap lane users.
6. These rules will be strictly enforced so all lap swimmers are able to get a workout.

Thank you for your cooperation, please notify the Member Services desk if you have any problems.

Figure 6-15. Posted pool rules.

DOCUMENTATION

When documenting hydrotherapy, specify what type of hydrotherapy was used and for what purpose. Note the patient's position or activities during the treatment session, as well as what level of assistance, if any, was needed. Note the water temperature if necessary as well as the water pressure and any additives to the water, if applicable. Be sure to include the duration of the treatment as well as the outcome or patient response.

See the following examples of documentation for hydrotherapy interventions.

Diagnosis: Patient has decreased muscle tone/movement in the left upper extremity post CVA.

O: Patient in therapy pool × 30 minutes, water 78°F, and performed left shoulder flexion/extension, abduction/adduction × 10 repetitions each and moderate assist. Also performed forward and backward walking × 10 minutes with use of upper extremities. Patient reported no increase in pain or discomfort during session.

Diagnosis: Patient with stage III pressure injury to sacrum.

O: Patient received pulsed lavage, 1000 mL warm saline, pressure 10 psi to stage III sacral pressure injury. Patient is right sidelying with area draped. Patient reported slight sensation of pressure but no discomfort. Wound measured at 5 × 3 × 0.8 cm before treatment session.

CONCLUSION

Hydrotherapy is a commonly used and beneficial modality to achieve specific physical therapy goals. One should be mindful of a patient's potential contraindications and adhere to safety precautions when using hydrotherapy.

While there are some limitations, such as cost, space, and infection control, hydrotherapy interventions offer options for therapists to address a variety of diagnoses.

REVIEW QUESTIONS

1. List and describe the physical properties of water.
2. Discuss how each physical property influences therapy interventions.
3. What are the physical therapy options for hydrotherapy interventions?
4. List the indications of hydrotherapy interventions.
5. Explain the contraindications for full-body immersion hydrotherapy.
6. What are the benefits of nonimmersion therapy vs localized or full-body immersion?
7. Discuss at least 3 safety or red flag concerns regarding hydrotherapy interventions.
8. Your patient has a severe left ankle sprain with 8/10 pain during range of motion activities. What hydrotherapy intervention would you recommend? How would you document that intervention?
9. Your patient has MS and presents with decreased endurance with overground gait. This patient uses a single-point cane for gait on the left. You would like to work on improving her endurance with gait. What hydrotherapy would you recommend? What should you be mindful of, given the MS diagnosis?

CASE STUDY 1

You are seeing a 72-year-old woman with a stage III pressure injury to her right calcaneus as a result of poor mobility after having a CVA 1 year ago. She does not complain of pain with the injury, and she does not ambulate except to transfer to the commode or wheelchair. The wound is 2 cm × 3.1 cm × 0.9 cm with granulation tissue noted from 12 o'clock to 4 o'clock but yellow slough from 4 o'clock to 11 o'clock. She has no tunneling or undermining, and exudate is thick and yellow. Your physical therapist wants you to work on cleaning out the wound to promote healing.

1. What hydrotherapy intervention would you recommend for this patient? Why?
2. What physiological effects would this intervention have on this patient's tissues?
3. What precautions should be taken when using hydrotherapy with this patient?
4. What other intervention(s) (not necessarily hydrotherapy) might you recommend? Why?
5. What nonmodality therapeutic activities/measures can be taken to help with wound healing?

CASE STUDY 2

You have a patient who is 48 years old and who had her knee replaced 8 weeks ago but has had continued pain and stiffness despite proper healing. Knee extension is -6 degrees and flexion is 96 degrees. She reports 6/10 pain with prolonged standing and walking, and she would like to be able to walk 1 mile around her neighborhood and resume gardening with less pain. She fatigues quickly and has decreased strength in that lower extremity. She also has difficulty climbing stairs. Your goal is to reduce the patient's pain while also improving her range of motion to 120 degrees of flexion and 0 degrees of extension and improving her strength.

1. What tissues are injured/affected?
2. What hydrotherapy intervention is appropriate for this patient? Why?
3. What are the contraindications for this intervention?
4. What are the parameters of this intervention?
5. What other (possibly nonhydrotherapy) interventions might be appropriate? Why?

REFERENCES

1. Volpe D, Giantin M, Maestri R, Frazzitta G. Comparing the effects of hydrotherapy and land-based therapy on balance in patients with Parkinson's disease: a randomized controlled pilot study. *Clin Rehabil*. 2014;28(12):1210-1217.
2. Cider A, Sveälv BG, Täng MS, Schaufelberger M, Andersson B. Immersion in warm water induces improvements in cardiac function in patients with chronic heart failure. *Eur J Heart Fail*. 2006;8(3):308-313.
3. Zamunér AR, Andrade CP, Forti M, et al. Effects of a hydrotherapy programme on symbolic and complexity dynamics of heart rate variability and aerobic capacity in fibromyalgia patients. *Clin Exp Rheumatol*. 2015;33(1 Suppl 88):S73-S81.
4. Hall J, Grant J, Blake D, Taylor G, Garbutt G. Cardiorespiratory responses to aquatic treadmill walking in patients with rheumatoid arthritis. *Physiother Res Int*. 2004;9(2):59-73.
5. Piotrowska-Całka E. Effects of a 24-week deep water aerobic training program on cardiovascular fitness. *Biol Sport*. 2010;27(2):95-98.
6. An J, Lee I, Yi Y. The thermal effects of water immersion on health outcomes: an integrative review. *Int J Environ Res Public Health*. 2019;16(7):1280-1301.
7. Held HE, Pendergrast, DR. Relative effects of submersion and increased pressure on respiratory mechanics, work, and energy cost of breathing. *J Appl Physiol (1985)*. 1985;114(5):578-591.
8. Thomaz S, Bernaldo P, Mateus S, Horan T, Leal JC. Effects of partial isothermic immersion on the spirometry parameters of tetraplegic patients. *Chest*. 2005;128(1):184-189.
9. Leal JC, Mateus SRM, Horan TA, Beraldo PSS. Effect of graded water immersion on vital capacity and plasma volume in patients with cervical spinal cord injury. *Spinal Cord*. 2010;48(5):375-379.
10. Sidiropoulou MP, Kokaridas DG, Giagazoglou PF, Karadonas MI, Fotiadou EG. Incidence of exercise-induced asthma in adolescent athletes under different training and environmental conditions. *J Strength Cond Res*. 2012;26(6):1644-1650.
11. Fitch KD, Morton AR. Specificity of exercise in exercise-induced asthma. *Br Med J*. 1971;4(5787):577-581.
12. Pechter U, Maaroos J, Mesikepp S, Veraksits A, Ots M. Regular low-intensity aquatic exercise improves cardiorespiratory functional capacity and reduces proteinuria in chronic renal failure patients. *Nephrol Dial Transplant*. 2003;18(3):624-625.
13. Becker BE. The biologic aspects of hydrotherapy. *J Back Musculoskelet Rehabil*. 1994;4(4):255-264.
14. Neville C, Henwood T, Beattie E, Fielding E. Exploring the effect of aquatic exercise on behavior and psychological well-being in people with moderate to severe dementia: a pilot study of the Watermemories Swimming Club. *Australas J Ageing*. 2014;33(2):124-127.
15. Acordi da Silva L, Tortelli L, Motta J, et al. Effects of aquatic exercise on mental health, functional autonomy and oxidative stress in depressed elderly individuals: a randomized clinical trial. *Clinics (Sao Paulo)*. 2019;74:e322.
16. American Physical Therapy Association. Choosing Wisely: five things physical therapist and patients should question. 2014. Accessed February 6, 2020. http://integrity.apta.org/ChoosingWisely/5Things/
17. Iannucci L. Making waves with aquatic therapy. *PT in Motion*. 2012;4(9):16-23.
18. Bastawros D. 5 things you need to know about: pulsed lavage. *Adv Skin Wound Care*. 2003;16(6):282.
19. Shetty R, Barreto E, Paul KM. Suction assisted pulse lavage: randomised controlled studies comparing its efficacy with conventional dressings in healing of chronic wounds. *Int Wound J*. 2014;11(1):55-63.
20. Centers for Disease Control and Prevention. Operating public hot tubs/spas. 2016. Accessed February 13, 2020. https://www.cdc.gov/healthywater/swimming/aquatics-professionals/operating-public-hot-tubs.html
21. American Physical Therapy Association. Marketplace. *PT: Magazine of Physical Therapy*. 1999;7(6):102.
22. Laskowski E. Water exercise: does pool temperature matter? 2018. Accessed February 13, 2020. https://www.mayoclinic.org/diseases-conditions/arthritis/expert-answers/water-exercise/faq-20057930
23. Giovanisci M. What is the perfect pool temperature? Swim University. 2019. Accessed February 13, 2020. https://www.swimuniversity.com/pool-temperature/
24. Tilden H, Mirsec M, Hutchinson B. Aquatic exercise programming for people with multiple sclerosis. 2003. Accessed February 13, 2020. https://www.nationalmssociety.org/NationalMSSociety/media/MSNationalFiles/Brochures/aquatic_exercise_program_03-16_v3.pdf
25. Centers for Disease Control and Prevention. Perceived exertion (Borg Rating of Perceived Exertion Scale). 1998. Accessed February 13, 2020. http://dhhs.ne.gov/ConcussionManage/Documents/BorgScaleExertion.pdf

Chapter 7

Traction

KEY TERMS Anulus fibrosus | Facet joints | Foramina | Intermittent | Intervertebral disc | Manual traction | Nucleus pulposus | Positional traction | Self-traction | Spinal nerve roots | Static

Chapter Objectives

1. Describe what traction is and the types of traction.
2. Discuss the physiological effects of traction.
3. Consider the ways traction is applied to physical therapy interventions.
4. Categorize the indications and contraindications for traction interventions.
5. Apply knowledge of traction set-up and parameters to case scenarios.
6. Document traction interventions correctly in a patient's chart.

Introduction

Traction is considered a mechanical energy modality that can be performed manually or with the use of traction machinery. One can also use gravity and body weight to generate a traction force. The goal of traction is to create a separation between 2 joint surfaces to relieve pain and improve function. Although this chapter will not discuss it specifically, traction is also used to promote fracture healing by holding bones and joints in proper alignment. This chapter will primarily focus on the use of spinal traction, although many of the principles can be applied to traction to the extremities.

To understand how traction works, one needs to remember basic anatomy of the spine. The spine is composed of 24 vertebrae stacked on top of each other connected by ligaments and surrounded by musculature. Between each bone is a vertebral disc that provides cushion and shock absorption. The disc has a soft center called a *nucleus pulposus* and a tough outer anulus fibrosus. The primary joints are the facet joints, and the spinal cord travels posterior to the vertebrae. There are exit points for spinal nerve roots, called *foramina*. Traction pulls apart the vertebrae, creating extra space for the vertebral discs and the nerves exiting out of the spinal cord. The ligaments, tendons, and muscles surrounding the vertebrae are also elongated during a traction force.

One should also remember that, like all other modalities, traction is not the sole answer to a patient's pain or dysfunction. Traction should be used as a means to progress a patient using other physical therapy interventions, but it should never be the only treatment for a patient.

Physiological Effects of Traction

To understand how traction yields decreased pain and improved function, one must first understand how traction affects the structures being pulled apart.

Memolo J.
Therapeutic Agents for the Physical Therapist Assistant
(pp 73-85). © 2022 SLACK Incorporated.

Nerve Impingement

As mentioned previously, the primary effect of traction is that it distracts, or pulls apart, joint surfaces. If the joint surfaces are too close together (or approximated), structures between the joints could become impinged and cause pain. The joints affected are most often facet joints, and the structures often affected by compression are the spinal nerve roots. If a patient complains of pain that radiates along an extremity, that is a good sign they may have some nerve impingement. A systematic review of studies determined that cervical traction (either mechanical or manual) decreased pain as a result of cervical radiculopathy when combined with other physical therapy interventions than with physical therapy alone.[1]

Disc Protrusion

Another structure that is often compressed by facet joints is the intervertebral disc. Compression causes the disc to protrude. The disc then loses its ability to provide sufficient cushion between the vertebrae, resulting in the bones drawing closer together.[2] The disc can bulge, and the soft nucleus pulposus may herniate, much like the jelly inside a doughnut squeezes out when the doughnut is compressed. This compression can result from repetitive actions, often from incorrect use of body mechanics with lifting or posture. A traction force that pulls apart the 2 vertebrae allows the disc to suck back into place, relieving pain.[3]

Stretching of Soft Tissue

Just as traction pulls apart joint surfaces, it also pulls on the soft tissue surrounding the joint. This applies to ligaments, tendons, and muscle tissue. Patients in pain may present with muscle guarding, which in turn causes more pain. The compression of soft tissue can also cause pain, and just as traction creates a space for nerves or discs, so too can the distraction of soft tissue.[4] As a result, pain may be reduced and range of motion (ROM) may be improved. These stretching effects are influenced both by the angle of pull as well as the load of pull.[3]

Joint Mobilization

Joint mobilization has been shown to decrease joint pain and increase ROM in joints. Manual joint mobilization can achieve these goals; however, manual joint mobilization typically focuses on one joint at a time. When using traction, multiple joints can be mobilized at the same time. In doing so, the mechanoreceptors in our tissues are stimulated, which may gate the pain sensations otherwise sent to the primary sensory cortex in the brain. Additionally, and possibly as another factor that decreases pain, traction may yield an improvement in joint ROM.[5]

Muscle Relaxation

If a patient is experiencing pain, they may not be able to fully relax. Muscle guarding, as mentioned previously, can create a pain cycle. A traction force can stretch and relax soft tissue, increase localized circulation, as well as provide space for nerves or discs to no longer be impinged, and any reduction of pain may yield relaxation. A study in 2017 measured muscle relaxation during inverted spinal traction by measuring electromyographic activity and determined that a 30- to 60-degree inversion angle yielded maximum muscle relaxation.[6] Both intermittent and static traction can yield a reduction in pain and thus muscle relaxation; many patients report relaxation during traction treatments, and it is not unusual to return at the end of a traction session to find a patient asleep on the table.

INDICATIONS AND CONTRAINDICATIONS OF TRACTION

Traction is a modality that has been in use since the days of ancient Rome,[7] and the benefits of it have been known despite the crude beginnings. However, as with all modalities, traction comes with its own dangers, and the contraindications for traction should be known and followed.

Indications for traction correlate to the physiological effects, so patients with nerve root impingement, herniated discs, decreased joint mobility (hypomobility), or muscle guarding or spasm would be excellent candidates for therapeutic traction.[8] As mentioned previously, herniated discs may be drawn back into the space between the vertebrae and create a space between the vertebrae with sustained traction. This can yield decreased pain from nerve root impingement, which in turn can result in decreased muscle guarding or spasm and improved joint mobility. Consult Box 7-1 for a research topic regarding the use of traction to improve herniated discs.

Despite these potential benefits, therapeutic traction comes with potential dangers to certain patient populations. Patients with joint hypermobility, for example, are not good candidates for traction. If the joint is already excessively mobile, adding additional mobility via traction

Table 7-1
Indications, Contraindications, and Physiological Effects of Therapeutic Traction

Indications	Contraindications	Physiological Effects
Disc herniation	Joint hypermobility	Reduction of nerve impingement
Joint hypomobility	Degenerative joint disease	Reduction of disc protrusion
Muscle guarding/spasm	Bone diseases (osteoporosis, arthritis, bone cancer)	Soft-tissue stretching
Nerve root impingement	Acute sprain, strain, inflammation	Joint mobilization
Connective tissue contractures	New peripheral or radicular nerve pain (stop traction)	Muscle relaxation
	Uncontrolled hypertension	Decreased pain
	Pregnancy	
	Aortic aneurysm	
	Claustrophobia (precaution)	
	Cough/sneezing (precaution)	
	Dentures (precaution)	
	Temporomandibular joint pain (precaution)	

can injure the joint. Similarly, if a patient is diagnosed with degenerative joint disease, pulling on those structures can further damage the joint. Bone-related diagnoses, such as osteoporosis, arthritis (especially rheumatoid), or cancer in the bone could make the bones themselves fragile and prone to fracture. Other contraindications include acute injuries such as sprains, strains, or joint inflammation, or any other injury or diagnosis for which joint movement is contraindicated. This might also include immediately postsurgery.

When a patient receives traction for nerve-related pain, which may present with pain radiating through an extremity, this pain should be relieved with traction forces. However, if a patient complains of new pain down the arms or legs, traction should be stopped immediately and one may need to assess the patient's sensation, motor function, or reflexes. This is because traction should decompress the nerve; peripheralization of pain through extremities or worsening of that pain means that decompression is not happening and one could further aggravate or prolong the injury.

Patients with uncontrolled hypertension may be contraindicated for traction because traction may cause an increase in blood pressure. Persons who are pregnant are usually contraindicated for traction because the traction belts compress the abdomen, and persons who are pregnant have lax joints due to the production of relaxin in preparation for childbirth. Pulling on these already lax joints could cause joint damage.

Traction is at least a precaution for patients who have claustrophobia because they may not enjoy being strapped to a table. If a patient has a cough or is sneezing, traction is also a precaution because a cough or sneeze during treatment could cause injury. If the patient is receiving cervical traction, patients with dentures or temporomandibular joint pain or dysfunction may be uncomfortable receiving traction. Table 7-1 lists the indications, contraindications, and physiological effects of traction.

APPLICATION METHODS

There are various ways to apply therapeutic traction to a patient. Much of this discussion will focus on mechanical traction; however, this chapter will address manual and positional traction techniques.

Mechanical Traction

When administering mechanical traction, the therapist uses a machine to create the traction force. The patient is frequently supine or prone on a traction table, with straps and belts connecting the patient to the table to pull on the affected area. Mechanical traction parameters include whether the traction force will be static (a sustained traction force the entire duration of treatment) or intermittent (the traction force cycles on and off), on and off times when using intermittent, the force of the pull (usually represented by pounds), treatment time, and the frequency of the treatment sessions. A clinic may have an old mechanical traction

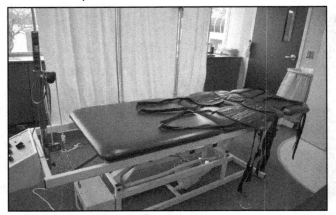

Figure 7-1. Older traction unit.

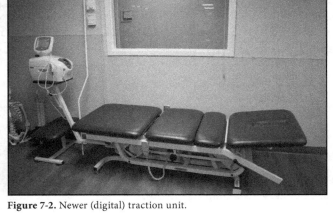

Figure 7-2. Newer (digital) traction unit.

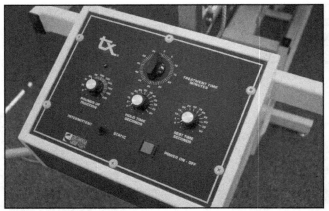

Figure 7-3. Older unit parameter screen.

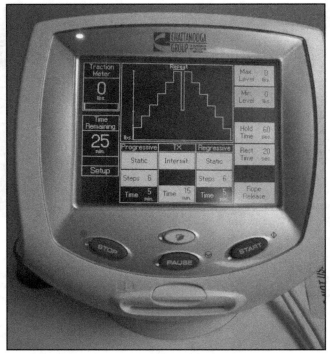

Figure 7-4. Newer unit parameter screen.

unit (Figure 7-1) or a newer model (Figure 7-2). The display screens also vary, as seen in Figure 7-3 for the older unit and Figure 7-4 for the digital unit. The settings for these parameters vary depending on whether one is administering lumbar or cervical traction and also on the rationale for treatment.

Mechanical Lumbar Traction

Newer research indicates there is no one set of parameters for lumbar mechanical traction.[9] However, Newton's laws show that to move a patient on a split table horizontally and overcome friction, as well as to separate the vertebrae, up to 50% of the patient's body weight must be used.[8] To cause changes in the space between vertebrae, some recommend 65 to 70 pounds of intermittent traction,[8] but the recommendations vary. Use of more than 400 pounds is considered excessive and injurious to the patient.

With regard to duration, the length of treatment may depend on the patient response or goal of treatment. For example, a relatively short time is required to treat a herniated disc. Traction forces that are too long can equalize the osmotic pressure between the disc and the surrounding tissues, losing the suction effect initially provided

by traction. Some studies suggest a treatment session of 10 to 15 minutes is sufficient to address a herniated disc,[8] whereas others recommend 8 to 10 minutes.[10] Also, if the traction is sustained or static, the duration is shorter than with intermittent traction. Other diagnoses with intermittent traction may need longer duration, up to 30 minutes. Some studies indicate a patient can tolerate more force with an intermittent traction set-up.[10]

Therapists administering intermittent traction will need to set the hold and relax, or on/off times, of the traction treatment. This is yet another parameter with changeable recommendations, but recent research indicates that a longer hold time (15 to 60 seconds) and shorter relax time (5 to 20 seconds) show the best improvement in lumbar

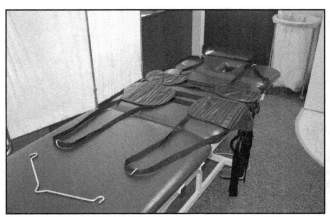

Figure 7-5. Lumbar straps set-up.

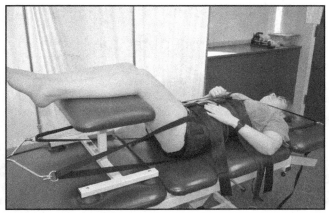

Figure 7-6. Patient on traction table strapped in.

ROM and pain.[11] Currently there is no definitive evidence that a particular frequency of treatment is more beneficial than another, although typical treatment parameters allow for 2 to 3 times weekly.[12] The frequency will again depend on the patient response and goals.

With respect to positioning, the patient will typically be in supine with the hips and knees flexed at 90 degrees over a stool or bolster. However, one can position the patient in prone in full extension. Prone might be best for patients who cannot tolerate supine or flexion, or who feel less discomfort in prone or extension. Prone might also be beneficial to posterior structures. Some studies indicate that prone positioning yields more immediate and more significant reduction in pain.[13] Most therapists set up the straps and belts before the patient gets on the table (Figure 7-5), and then position the patient on the table to align with the belts. One needs thoracic and pelvic nonslip belts that will connect to the top and the bottom of the table. When securing the patient to the table, the belts need to be tight enough to prevent the patient from sliding out of the belts or being pulled up the table. Figure 7-6 shows a patient strapped into a traction table.

Typically, lumbar traction is administered bilaterally, meaning the pull is equal on both sides; however, if symptoms are unilateral, traction can be set up for a unilateral pull. The angle of pull can be adjusted; there is no agreed-on angle of pull to yield specific results at this time, and most studies indicate that determining the angle of pull is determined by patient response. Some research indicates that the higher the degree of lumbar flexion, the higher lumbar spine segments are affected, and the less lumbar flexion, the lower lumbar spine segments are affected.[8]

If a patient is benefitting from lumbar traction, you or the physical therapist may recommend the use of a home lumbar traction unit (Figure 7-7). Home lumbar traction units come in transportable bags and can be set up easily on the floor or a firm bed surface. The patient will be strapped into the device and can set the force using a connected pump. These devices can be pricey, however, and it

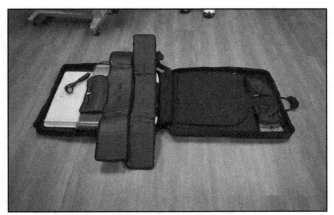

Figure 7-7. Home lumbar unit.

is important to confirm that the patient understands how to set the parameters on the unit so as not to cause injury. Table 7-2 details the set-up and parameters for mechanical lumbar traction.

Mechanical Cervical Traction

Mechanical cervical traction can be set up similarly to mechanical lumbar traction. One may use a traction table, set up for a cervical intervention, or one can use a home cervical traction unit.

Whereas mechanical lumbar traction allows for prone or supine positioning, mechanical cervical traction is performed in supine. A sitting position is usually not recommended because it is difficult for the patient to fully relax in this position. One may see over-the-door halters, but these are not generally recommended for safe cervical traction because they can injure a person's jaw and are difficult to set up because of the angle and force of the pull.

In supine, the patient will benefit from having a bolster under the knees to decrease pressure on the back and the head placed in the halter. When applying cervical traction, consider the angle of flexion with the machine; most clinicians recommend 20 to 30 degrees of flexion, which will

Table 7-2	
Procedures for Applying Mechanical Lumbar Traction	
Equipment Needed	• Split traction table and traction unit OR portable lumbar traction unit • Thoracic and pelvic belts • Stool or bolster • Rope and spreader bar
Treatment/ Parameters	• Confirm patient does not have contraindications. • Select appropriate traction device. • Determine optimal patient position—prone or supine. • Set up belts on traction table; if using portable unit, set up unit on firm surface and set up belts. • Ensure table (if a split table) is locked at this point. • Position patient on table or unit and align with belts; attach and tighten the belts to patient. Belts are ideally placed directly on patient's skin. • Connect belts to traction table; position patient's lower extremities on stool (if in supine) to create 90-90 position. • Set the traction parameters: static/intermittent, poundage (50% of body weight to separate vertebrae). If using portable unit, show patient how to release pressure if needed. • Unlock split table and start traction; let machine run through 2 to 3 cycles to ensure harnesses are holding and patient is comfortable—make changes if necessary. • Provide patient a call bell and emergency shutoff button; make sure patient understands when to use this button. • When treatment is complete, stop traction and assess patient's response. • Lock table back to a closed position, release tension in harness straps first, and allow patient to lie still for a moment before removing harnesses. Have patient sit up slowly and sit at the edge of the table for another few moments before standing or walking.
Safety Considerations	• Monitor patient during first few cycles of treatment and then again after treatment is complete. • Be ready to adjust or change interventions depending on patient response. • Provide patient a call bell and emergency shutoff button and ensure patient is educated on use. • Release tension slowly in traction and harnesses; make patient lie and sit for a few moments to avoid dizziness or falling.
Advantages	• Mechanical traction provides more force to yield improved results with pain and mobility • Parameters can be easily set to adjust to patient response and outcomes • Portable units easy for patient to set up and use at home
Disadvantages	• Level of difficulty with setting up machine and harnesses • Risk of increased pain depending on parameters used • Machine large, expensive • Portable units expensive, potential for patient to set up incorrectly

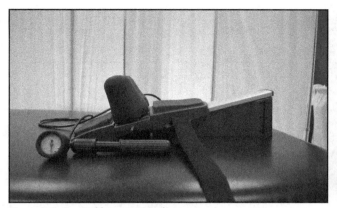

Figure 7-8. Cervical home unit and pump.

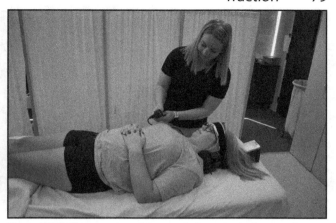

Figure 7-9. Patient set-up receiving cervical traction on home unit.

affect the posterior structures of the cervical spine, while an extended position affects the anterior structures and disc spaces.[14] As with lumbar traction, cervical traction is often administered bilaterally, but it can be adjusted to pull unilaterally if the patient displays or complains of unilateral pain.

Mechanical cervical traction can be applied statically (or sustained) or intermittently. Indications for sustained vs intermittent traction include disc herniations, muscle spasms, or soft-tissue tightness.[15] Intermittent traction has a hold-and-relax setting, just as with lumbar traction, and typically, intermittent traction is applied for a longer duration than sustained.

Just as lumbar traction requires a minimal weight to overcome body weight and friction, so does cervical traction. Clinicians suggest that 10 pounds of force is necessary to overcome the weight of the head and separate the atlantoaxial and atlantooccipital joints, that 11 to 15 pounds can stretch tight tissue or address muscle spasms, and that 20 to 30 pounds is required to separate the rest of the cervical vertebrae.[15] Cervical traction force should begin small and incrementally be increased as long as the patient has no complaints. One should not exceed 45 pounds for cervical traction.[15]

As with lumbar traction, there are home cervical traction units (Figure 7-8). Patients should be thoroughly educated on how to set up the unit, and they may need some assistance from a caregiver with strapping into the unit. First, the angle of pull is adjusted according to what part of the cervical spine is being addressed. The patient will then lie supine with the head positioned so the bolsters are just under the occiput. The patient's head is strapped in, and then the patient can use the hand pump to increase the force of pull. Most units max out at 50 pounds. Figure 7-9 shows a patient set-up on a home cervical traction unit. Table 7-3 details the set-up and parameters for mechanical cervical traction.

Manual Traction

Mechanical traction is not appropriate for a patient when the force is too great, or the patient is uncomfortable being strapped onto a table. Perhaps the therapist's clinic does not own a traction table or portable traction units. In these cases, manual traction can be a useful option. Manual traction is performed when the therapist uses their hands or sometimes other tools to pull joint surfaces apart. The force of pull with manual traction is far less than what a table can provide; however, many patients enjoy and benefit from manual traction interventions.[16]

Lumbar manual traction is often performed with the patient in supine or sometimes a hooklying position. There are a variety of manual traction methods, and this text cannot cover all possibilities; however, it will attempt to discuss some of the more popular or common methods. One such method is for the therapist to pull on the patient's leg. This is typically performed unilaterally, and the force of pull is dependent on the patient's response as well as whether the patient is secured to the treatment table. Figure 7-10 shows a patient receiving a unilateral leg pull. If the patient is secured, more force can be applied without pulling the patient off the table. The therapist can adjust the amount of force used according to patient response, although the force amount is often unmeasured unless the therapist uses a force gauge. Patient-reported measures, then, are typically the determinant of success with this treatment.

If the patient requires a bilateral pull, the patient can be in a hooklying position (Figure 7-11), and the therapist pulls on the lower extremities (LEs) from behind the knees bilaterally. Another technique is to have the patient lie supine with their legs on a therapy ball. The therapist can then opt from a variety of choices. The therapist can pull on the patient's knees to create a distraction force (Figure 7-12). This option does not generate a significant amount of force, so another option is to use a series of gait belts strapped around the patient and then around the therapist so the therapist can use their own body weight to apply more force. Figure 7-13 shows this type of manual traction technique. The amount of force generated can be increased, as with the unilateral pull example, if the patient is secured to the treatment table. Gait belts or straps are often used during manual traction therapy because of the repetitive strain

Table 7-3	
Procedures for Applying Mechanical Cervical Traction	
Equipment Needed	• Traction table and traction unit OR portable lumbar traction unit • Cervical traction halter • Stool or bolster • Rope and spreader bar
Treatment/ Parameters	• Confirm patient does not have contraindications. • Select appropriate traction device. • Determine optimal patient position—supine is most common. • Set up cervical harness on traction table; if using portable unit, set up unit on firm surface and adjust angle. • Make sure split table is locked at this point. Position patient on table or portable unit and set up in halter. • Connect halter to traction table. • Set up traction parameters, including static/intermittent and poundage (10 lb initially; 11 to 15 lb for soft-tissue stretch, and 20 to 30 lb for vertebral separation). If using a portable unit, show patient how to release pressure if needed. • Begin traction treatment; let the unit run through 2 to 3 cycles before leaving patient alone to ensure harnesses work correctly and patient is comfortable. Make changes if necessary. • When treatment is complete, stop traction and assess patient's response. • Lock table back and have the patient lie still for a few moments when harnesses/tension are released. Have patient sit up slowly and sit for a few moments to prevent dizziness or falling.
Safety Considerations	• Monitor patient during first few cycles of the treatment and then again after treatment is complete. • Be ready to adjust or change interventions depending on patient response. • Provide patient a call bell and emergency cutoff button; make sure the patient is educated on how and when to use this button. • Release tension slowly in traction and harnesses; make patient lie and then sit for a few moments to avoid dizziness or falling.
Advantages	• Mechanical traction provides more force to yield improved results with pain and mobility • Parameters can be easily set to adjust to patient response and outcomes • Portable units easy for patient to set up and use at home
Disadvantages	• Level of difficulty with setting up machine and harnesses • Risk of increased pain depending on parameters used • Machine large, expensive • Portable units expensive, potential for patient to set up incorrectly

on therapists' hands and body; these allow the therapist to maintain the traction force longer without as much fatigue.

Manual cervical traction also makes use of both the therapist's hands and tools to facilitate a greater force and a longer duration of treatment. Manual cervical traction typically occurs with the patient placed in supine with the LEs supported by a bolster or towel roll. Therapist body mechanics are best when they can be seated at the patient's head and are able to place their arms on the treatment table for support. The therapist lifts and cradles the patient's head with their hands, finding the occiput as the landmark to provide the traction pull (Figure 7-14). As with the lumbar manual traction, the pull can be adjusted according to the patient response and outcomes. Manual therapy such

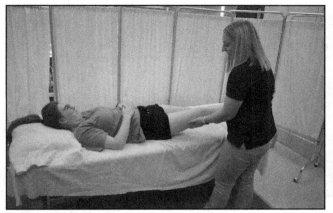

Figure 7-10. Patient receiving unilateral leg pull.

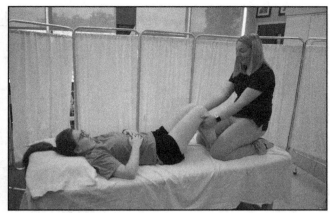

Figure 7-11. Hooklying patient, with therapist pulling from behind knees.

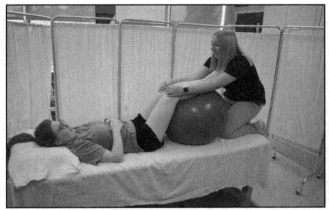

Figure 7-12. Patient with LEs over swiss ball while therapist pulls at knees.

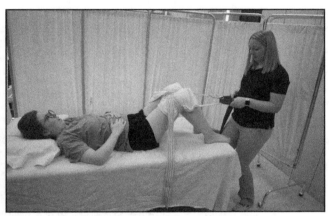

Figure 7-13. Patient with therapist using gait belts to pull.

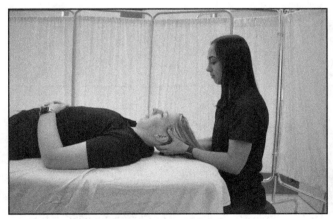

Figure 7-14. Manual cervical traction with hands.

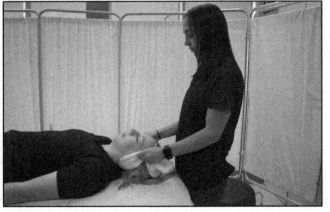

Figure 7-15. Manual cervical traction with pillow case.

as soft-tissue mobilization is often combined with manual cervical traction, and the patient's head can also be rotated to the left and right to create distraction forces unilaterally. While lumbar traction requires more force in some cases, cervical traction usually does not. If the therapist's hands fatigue, they can use a pillow case, towel roll, or gait belt around the patient's head (secured to provide the pull at the patient's occiput) as a means to pull. Figure 7-15 shows this adaptation for a manual pull.

Keep in mind that there are other options for manual therapy that will be discussed in a later chapter. Table 7-4 provides the specifics on how to provide manual traction.

Table 7-4		
Procedures for Applying Manual Lumbar and Cervical Traction		
Equipment Needed	• Therapist, patient • Towel, pillow case, gait belt, therapy ball (as needed)	
Treatment/ Parameters	• Confirm patient does not have contraindications. • Determine optimal patient position—supine or hooklying are most common. If traction table and harnesses are available, you may want to secure patient to table. • For lumbar traction: therapist is positioned at patient's feet/LEs. Position hands behind patient's knees and apply traction. Alternately, position patient's LEs over a therapy ball and pull with hands, or use a gait belt to pull (with or without therapy ball). • For cervical traction: therapist is positioned at patient's head, ideally seated to promote improved body mechanics. Place supinated hands under patient's head with forearms resting on treatment table; fingers should palpate for the occiput. Apply traction by pulling with hands; alternately, use a towel roll, pillow case, or gait belt to provide additional force. • When treatment is complete, stop traction and assess patient's response. • Traction can be applied intermittently or statically, depending on what the therapist can do and how patient responds to treatment.	
Safety Considerations	• Monitor patient's response (verbally and visually) during treatment session; adjust treatment accordingly. • Initiate and release tension slowly in traction; make patient lie and then sit for a few moments to avoid dizziness or falling.	
Advantages	• Little to no equipment required • Little to no set-up time required • Force can be manually adjusted according to patient feedback • Ideal for patients who cannot tolerate stronger forces of mechanical traction, who have contraindications for mechanical traction, or who cannot tolerate harnesses of mechanical traction	
Disadvantages	• Traction force is limited by therapist strength and endurance • Difficulty with accurately or objectively measuring and documenting traction force • Requires a skilled clinician to apply	

Positional Traction

A patient may need traction at home, and yet is unable to afford or have access to a home mechanical unit. There are positional traction techniques a patient can learn to receive safe traction at home. While positional traction applies even less force than manual traction, and much less force than mechanical traction, it can provide a prolonged stretch of shortened tissues and allow for relaxation in the case of muscle spasm. Again, there are a variety of options for positional traction, but a few of the most representative choices will be listed here.

One easy choice for bilateral lower back pain is to have the patient perform bilateral knee-to-chest positioning. The patient begins in supine and pulls their knees to the chest and holds that position; the patient can repeat this several times to relieve pain. Figure 7-16 provides an example of this position. This positioning is optimal to yield an increase in the size of the lumbar foramen bilaterally. If a unilateral position is required, patients can position themselves in sidelying with the painful side up over a towel roll, folded pillow, or small bolster between the iliac crest and the rib cage (Figure 7-17).[17] The patient can also flex their knees to create lumbar flexion, which can further open up the foramina. The patient can stay in this position for a prolonged period to decrease pain.

Other positional traction techniques include the use of an inversion traction unit, which puts a strapped-in patient in an inverted, or upside-down, position. Gravity will do the work of pulling the vertebrae apart. A patient can also use a kitchen counter corner or a chair (Figure 7-18), to let gravity help, or a patient can hang from an overhead bar to let gravity pull the vertebrae apart.

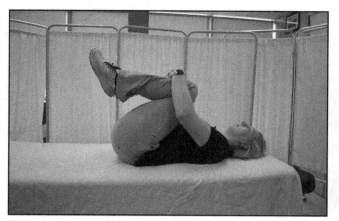

Figure 7-16. Knee-to-chest position.

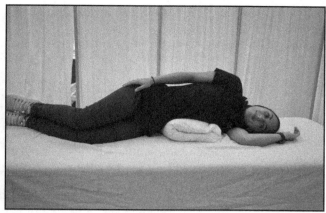

Figure 7-17. Sidelying over towel roll.

SAFETY CONCERNS

When treating a patient with mechanical or manual traction, it is important to consider the safety steps and concerns one must follow to provide an effective and safe treatment. For example, if a patient is receiving mechanical traction, and is thusly secured to a treatment table with the therapist possibly away from the patient, the patient must be provided the safety cutoff switch or button. This button will slowly stop the traction and release the force (it is important that this happens slowly so as to not cause the muscles to spasm). The patient should be educated about the use of this button; the patient would use it if experiencing new or worsening pain, if they feel the need to cough or sneeze, or if the patient is otherwise uncomfortable. Additionally, the patient should be provided some sort of call button or bell to gain the therapist's attention.

As mentioned previously, the tension of any traction force should be released, and for that matter, initiated gradually. A sudden start or stop of traction could yield increased pain or muscle spasm. Most traction machines will build up and release force gradually, and the therapist should stay in the treatment area to ensure this is the case before leaving the patient alone. Even when the emergency release button is pressed, mechanical traction units will release the tension gradually. When a traction session is complete and the tension is released, the patient should first have the straps of the harness loosened (but not yet removed) to allow the muscles to relax slowly. After a few minutes, the harness can then be unclipped and removed.

Once unstrapped from the table, the patient should be instructed to sit up slowly and to sit at the edge of the treatment table for another few minutes before standing and moving. The patient has been in a supine or prone position for up to 30 minutes, and may experience dizziness on sitting.

For patients considering the use of positional traction, particularly inversion traction, those with uncontrolled hypertension, heart disease, or glaucoma should be

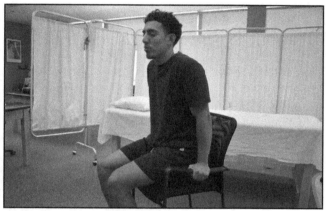

Figure 7-18. Chair with push up.

monitored closely. The change in position can affect blood pressure, and those with uncontrolled hypertension may experience dizziness, vertigo, or nausea, or may otherwise exacerbate the symptoms of inversion positioning. In cases like this, at-home treatment would be contraindicated.

DOCUMENTATION

When documenting traction, note what type of traction was used (mechanical, manual, positional) and then specify what area (lumbar or cervical) was treated. The therapist can, of course, be more specific to what spinal level was addressed, and for the purpose of the treatment, one can indicate the diagnosis and/or the goal (eg, to decrease pain, to increase ROM). As with all modality interventions, every parameter should be listed, including whether the traction was applied in an intermittent or static form, for how long, with what force, bilaterally or unilaterally, and so on. Be sure to document the patient's positioning as well as the patient's response to the treatment. If the patient had to stop the session because of increased pain or worsening symptoms, this would be included in the documentation.

The following examples should help give an idea of how to document a traction session.

Diagnosis: Patient is in therapy because of bilateral lower back pain (7/10) resulting in decreased mobility, strength, and endurance.

O: Reviewed contraindications with patient. Patient received lower lumbar spine mechanical traction using mechanical traction table. Patient positioned in supine with LEs elevated to 90-90 position using stool. Patient received 55 pounds of force intermittently for 50:10 seconds × 8 minutes. Patient reported pain at 5/10 after treatment session and had no other complaints.

Diagnosis: Patient being seen by therapy status post car accident with whiplash injury 8 weeks ago. Patient continues to have pain in cervical spine (6/10), worse by the end of the day. Patient is cleared by physician to receive manual cervical traction.

O: Reviewed contraindications with patient. Patient positioned in supine with bolster under knees for comfort. Patient received static bilateral manual cervical traction × 10 minutes with therapist using gait belt. Patient reported pain at 3/10 after therapy session with no other complaints.

Conclusion

Traction can decrease pain and increase mobility by distracting joint spaces, relaxing muscles, or stretching soft tissues. This can be performed mechanically, manually, or positionally, and each method can be tailored to the patient's diagnosis and needs. Contraindications for traction should be known and reviewed with patients before treatment, but barring these, traction can provide significant relief for many patients.

Review Questions

1.   What are the different types of traction?
2.   How would one make the clinical judgment of using one type of traction over another?
3.   What are the physiological effects of traction?
4.   List the indications for using traction with a patient.
5.   Discuss one technique for applying manual lumbar traction to your patient.
6.   Discuss the safety concerns or set-up for mechanical lumbar or cervical traction.
7.   List the contraindications for traction.

8.   What is the maximum force one can apply (mechanically) for lumbar traction? What about for cervical traction?
9.   You have a patient with unilateral lower lumbar pain, 7/10. What options do you have for traction interventions? Be specific about set-up.
10. Your patient received mechanical cervical traction for 10 minutes with a 20-pound force statically while in supine. Document the "O" section for this treatment session.

Case Study 1

Your patient is a 58-year-old man with cervical pain after doing drywall repair and painting in his house 3 days ago. Imaging shows no injury to the discs, but the patient does have cervical and upper trapezius pain rated at 4/10 and up to 7/10 when he extends his neck. ROM is normal but painful at the end range. Your physical therapy goal is to decrease pain to allow for pain-free ROM.

1.   What tissues are injured/affected?
2.   What traction intervention would you recommend? Why?
3.   What parameters would you follow for this intervention?
4.   What are the physiological effects of traction?
5.   What other modalities would be appropriate for this patient? Why?

Case Study 2

Your patient is a 49-year-old man who works as a lineman but has begun to have radiating pain originating at L5. Pain is rated at 6/10, especially when he attempts to bend over or with prolonged sitting. Lying down is currently the only thing that relieves his pain. He reports no numbness or tingling, just pain. The pain radiates down into his right thigh and calf. He has limited forward flexion ROM because of pain, but sensation and reflexes all intact. The plan is to reduce the patient's pain to promote full ROM and return function.

1.   What are the tissues affected?
2.   What traction intervention would you recommend? Why?
3.   What are the parameters you would recommend?
4.   What are the contraindications for this intervention?
5.   What other therapeutic interventions would you suggest for this patient? Why?

References

1. Romeo A, Vanti C, Boldrini V, et al. Cervical radiculopathy: effectiveness of adding traction to physical therapy—a systematic review and meta-analysis of randomized controlled trials. *Phys Ther.* 2018;98(4):231-242.

2. Karimi N, Akbarov P, Rahnama L. Effects of segmental traction therapy on lumbar disc herniation in patients with acute low back pain measured by magnetic resonance imaging: a single arm clinical trial. *J Back Musculoskelet Rehabil.* 2017;30(2):247-253.

3. Farajpour H, Jamshidi N. Effects of different angles of the traction table on lumbar spine ligaments: a finite element study. *Clin Orthop Surg.* 2017;9(4):480-488.

4. Nishigami T, Ikeuchi M, Okanoue Y, et al. A pilot feasibility study for immediate relief of referred knee pain by hip traction in hip osteoarthritis. *J Orthop Sci.* 2012;17(3):328-330.

5. Creighton DS, Marsh D, Gruca M, Walter M. The application of a pre-positioned upper cervical traction mobilization to patients with painful active cervical rotation impairment: a case series. *J Back Musculoskelet Rehabil.* 2017;30(5):1053-1059.

6. Kang J, Hyong I. Changes in electromyographic activity of lumbar paraspinal muscled according to type of inverted-spinal-traction. *Wirel Pers Commun.* 2017;93(1):35-45.

7. Shterenshis MV. The history of modern spinal traction with particular reference to neural disorders. *Spinal Cord.* 1997;35(3):139-146.

8. Saunders HD. Lumbar traction. *J Orthop Sports Phys Ther.* 1979;1(1):36-45.

9. Alrwaily M, Almurtiri M, Schneider M. Assessment of variability in traction interventions for patients with low back pain: a systematic review. *Chiropr Man Therap.* 2018;26(1):35.

10. Pellecchia G. Lumbar traction: a review of the literature. *J Orthop Sports Phys Ther.* 1994;20(5):262-267.

11. Santhumayor R, Kumar D, Ajith S. Effects of four different hold and rest time combinations of intermittent lumbar traction in the treatment of lumbar intervertebral disc prolapse: a comparative study. *Int J Health Sci Res.* 2015;6(1):214-220.

12. Harte AA, Gracey JH, Baxter GD. Current use of lumbar traction in the management of low back pain: results of a survey of physiotherapists in the United Kingdom. *Arch Phys Med Rehabil.* 2005;86(6):1164-1169.

13. Filiz MB, Kiliç Z, Uçkun A, et al. Mechanical traction for lumbar radicular pain: supine or prone? A randomized controlled trial. *Am J Phys Med Rehabil.* 2018;97(6):433-439.

14. Harris PR. Cervical traction: review of literature and treatment guidelines. *Phys Ther.* 1977;57(8):910-914.

15. University of Western States. WSCC Clinics. Cervical traction. 2008. Accessed March 21, 2020. https://ftp.uws.edu/udocs/public/CSPE_Protocols_and_Care_Pathways/Protocols/Cervical_Traction.pdf

16. Oh H, Choi S, Lee S, Choi J, Lee K. The impact of manual spinal traction therapy on the pain and Oswestry disability index of patients with chronic back pain. *J Phys Ther Sci.* 2018;30(12):1455-1457.

17. Creighton DS. Positional distraction, a radiological confirmation. *J Man Manip Ther.* 1993;1(3):83-86.

Chapter 8

Compression

KEY TERMS Deep vein thrombosis | Edema | Erythema | Hydrostatic pressure | Intermittent | Long-stretch bandage | Lymphatic fluid | Lymphedema | Osmotic pressure | Resting pressure | Short-stretch bandage | Static | Venous stasis ulcer | Working pressure

KEY ABBREVIATIONS CHF | DVT

CHAPTER OBJECTIVES

1. Understand what compression is and the different types of compression.
2. Discuss the physiological effects of compression.
3. Consider the ways compression is applied to physical therapy interventions.
4. Categorize the indications and contraindications for compression interventions.
5. Apply knowledge of compression set-up and parameters to case scenarios.
6. Document compression interventions correctly in a patient's chart.

INTRODUCTION

Anyone who has ever sprained an ankle or wrist probably was told to follow the RICE procedure: rest, ice, compression, and elevation. In an earlier chapter, the benefits of ice were detailed in order to address pain and swelling. Compression is another way to reduce edema and its associated pain. However, compression is not used only for edema. A physical therapist assistant can use compression to shape a residual limb after a patient has had an amputation; it can prevent deep vein thromboses (DVTs), which could become emboli that travel to the heart, brain, or lungs; it

can be used as a component of wound healing; and it can be used to decrease or modify scar tissue. Compression can be either static (with constant pressure during the treatment) or intermittent (with the pressure on and off per a set of parameters) and the decision of which type a therapist uses will depend on the goals of the treatment.

PHYSIOLOGICAL EFFECTS OF COMPRESSION

Compression's physiological effects include effects on circulation as well as tissue size and shape. First circulation will be discussed.

Effects on Circulation

Edema can be caused by an injury, such as the aforementioned sprained ankle. When one sustains an injury, the healing process begins, and this is initiated by the inflammation phase of healing. The body works to stop the bleeding (if bleeding is occurring), and it sends white blood cells, enzymes, nutrients, as well as macrophages and neutrophils to the area. The injury itself has caused damage to the cells, and fluids collect in the interstitial spaces. The classic signs of inflammation, such as erythema (redness), edema, warmth, and pain, are noted in the area. While the inflammation phase is necessary for effective healing, the excessive pain and loss of function associated with it can be mitigated by using compression.

Memolo J.
Therapeutic Agents for the Physical Therapist Assistant
(pp 87-98). © 2022 SLACK Incorporated.

Box 8-1

Box 8-1

Research Topic

Consider whether the use of pneumatic compression is superior to the use of compression garments/stockings in the prevention of DVTs after surgery. What does the research say on this topic? Develop a patient, intervention, comparison, outcome, time question to help address this topic.

Compression affects the hydrostatic pressure in the tissues, which in turn increases the local circulation. Think about the earlier conversation about hydrostatic pressure as generated by water. Compression is no different. In this case, hydrostatic pressure is affected by gravity, blood pressure, and the effects of inflammation. In a normal, healthy body, hydrostatic pressure works to push fluid out of the blood vessels and osmotic pressure works to keep the fluid in the blood vessels balanced. However, when an injury or some other malfunction occurs, this balance is disrupted and lymphatic fluid collects in the interstitial spaces, and when this happens, the fluid deforms the surrounding tissue and causes pain. Coupled with the effects of gravity (a more dependent portion of the body will see more edema because gravity makes it difficult to move upward), this change in balance yields increased swelling. Compression can increase the hydrostatic pressure in the interstitial spaces and, in doing so, cause fluid to be drawn back into the lymphatic vessels. Compression creates circulation that moves the excess fluid up toward the heart to be recirculated throughout the body by compressing the vessels and moving the fluid proximally.[1] Elevation of the body part also assists with this process because it helps to overcome gravity's effects. One might also suggest a patient perform ankle pumps or other exercises, as the muscle contraction can move fluid upward.

By moving this fluid so that it does not linger in the extremities, one can potentially prevent a DVT from forming. Box 8-1 offers a research opportunity on this topic. Similarly, venous stasis ulcers, which may form as a result of or a complication from edema in a limb, can heal faster if the edema is reduced.

Effects on Tissue Size and Shape

Compression can be used to alter the shape or size of tissue, specifically scar tissue or a residual limb.

Scarring is a normal part of the healing process. Depending on the type of injury and the length of time healing took, a scar can be neat and barely noticeable, whereas others can be pronounced. Wounds that heal by first intention (ie, via sutures, staples, or glue) usually yield small, neat scars that may be difficult to see. However, most people have at least one scar that must heal by second

intention. These wounds have irregular edges that cannot be approximated, so some other form of wound care must occur, and these wounds can result in more noticeable scars. Some scars can be the result of extensive injuries. Consider a person who has experienced burns over large portions of their body. These burn scars may be raised, red, and likely will not be very malleable, meaning that the patient will have limited range of motion (ROM) in those areas if the scar tissue is not addressed. Some people scar extensively even with minor cuts or injuries. Keloid scars are those that spread beyond the boundaries of the original wound.[2] They invade normal surrounding skin and are difficult to eradicate even with excision. Hypertrophic scars are raised scars, but they stay within the boundaries of the original wound. They can be red, inflamed, and sometimes itchy.[2] Compression can be used as a means to prevent the formation of raised or extensive scarring. Patients who have experienced burns often wear custom garments over that area (more on this later) to compress and form the scar tissue. Someone who is prone to keloid or hypertrophic scars may also benefit from compression wraps, garments, or silicone gel sheets to decrease the scarring.[3] A compression wrap is a noninvasive method, and because it is very tight and elastic, mimicking normal skin, it flattens the scar. This means the scar may not grow as much or at all, and if a scar does form, it may be lighter, softer, less thick, and less uncomfortable than without the compression.[4] Another type of compression, silicone gel sheets, are often used to decrease scarring. While the exact mechanism for how these work is uncertain, the hypothesis is that they occlude the scar site and hydrate the wound bed, suppressing the overactivity of scar-related cells and thus decreasing scarring.[5] These sheets can be reusable or in a single-use format that reduce the risk of infection. They are also lower in cost and can easily be used at home.[5] Compression can also facilitate improved ROM.[4]

Similarly, compression can positively affect sensitivity and formation of residual limbs. When a person undergoes an amputation, the residual limb is somewhat squared off. A skin flap is folded over the edge of the bone and stapled in place. If a person desires to wear a prosthetic limb, the residual limb will need to be shaped to fit the prosthetic socket; the socket is typically a conical shape. Once a person has had the amputation surgery and the wound has healed, they immediately begin a regimen of wearing either wraps or a garment (or both) to begin shaping the residual limb. The garments fit precisely to the limb and reduce edema as well as encourage the limb into the conical shape required for the prosthesis.[6] A prosthetist works closely with the patient to measure and order new garments as the residual limb shrinks and shapes. A physical therapist assistant will often be one of the communicators with the prosthetist and will provide education and assistance to patients as they learn how to don the garment. If wraps are used, the physical therapist assistant can apply those wraps.

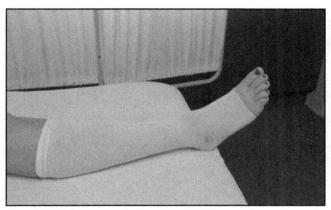

Figure 8-1. Thromboembolic deterrant (TED) hose.

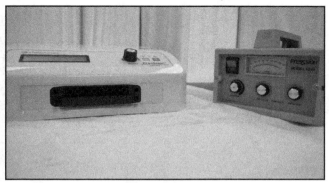

Figure 8-2. Intermittent compression units.

It is not uncommon for people with amputations to suffer from phantom pains in the removed limb. If the left lower extremity was removed, patients may feel like their left big toe hurts or have pain in the knee, even if they no longer have a knee. Sometimes, individuals feel sensations like an itch in a limb that is no longer there. Although it is unclear exactly what causes phantom limb pain, most think it has something to do with receiving mixed signals from the brain; the brain does not yet recognize that the limb is gone, and the missing input from that limb yields a painful or abnormal sensation, possibly due to a rewiring of peripheral nerves.[7] Because compression garments fit very closely with the skin, they help send signals to the brain that the limb ends in this new location and there is no big toe to itch or knee to hurt.[8]

INDICATIONS AND CONTRAINDICATIONS OF COMPRESSION

As mentioned previously, one of the primary physiological effects of compression is its ability to control edema. Therefore, any diagnosis that is accompanied by edema is a clinical indication for compression. If the patient has incurred an acute injury, such as a sprained or strained ankle, wrist, knee, elbow, or any other body part, compression in the form of a wrap could be helpful.

There are, of course, other causes for edema. Often it has something to do with venous or lymphatic insufficiency, meaning that either the veins or the lymphatic vessels (or both) have difficulty with or are unable to pump fluid toward the heart. Some people notice their lower extremities swell during or shortly after an airplane ride. Many individuals who are pregnant experience swollen lower extremities, especially as their pregnancies progress, which is attributed to increased blood volume, hormonal effects on venous smooth muscles, and increased pressure in the veins caused by the growing uterus. People who have congestive heart failure (CHF), diabetes, or acute renal disease may have edema as well.

Lymphedema is a condition in which there is decreased lymphatic flow, often due to damage or malfunction of the lymphatic vessels and/or the lymph nodes. Normally, lymph fluid travels through the lymph vessels and nodes and empty into the subclavian vein, where the kidneys process it to eliminate waste products. A person with lymphedema may have incurred some injury to lymph vessels or nodes, meaning that the fluid that normally moves freely around the body collects in a specific area. The primary cause of primary lymphedema is generally congenital; however, most lymphedema cases result from secondary causes, including infection, cancer, radiation therapy, surgery, and trauma.[9]

Another indication for compression is the prevention of DVTs. These blood clots are potentially dangerous because they can be dislodged and move from the deep vein to another part of the body and cause a cerebrovascular accident, myocardial infarction, or pulmonary embolism. Risk factors for DVTs include postsurgery status, immobility, advanced age, cancer, pacemakers, use of oral contraceptives, pregnancy, and hormone therapy. Clinicians can often observe when a DVT is present by noting the classic signs of inflammation, including swelling in the area, warmth in the area, and pain or discomfort with movement or palpation. Patients who are at risk for DVT formation may be advised to wear external compression stockings (Figure 8-1). Some evidence shows that wearing compression stockings when flying on an airplane can reduce the occurrence of edema and also the risk for DVT formation.[10] While most clinicians agree that external stockings are a reliable prophylaxis for DVT formation, there is conflicting evidence to support this claim,[11] and another study showed that the use of compression stocking to prevent postthrombotic syndrome is ineffectual.[12] There was a study that compared the use of knee-high vs thigh-high stockings and determined that the thigh-high stocking better prevented DVTs.[13]

Alternately, many hospitals favor the use of intermittent compression to prevent DVTs, but again, the research varies. Figure 8-2 shows a typical intermittent compression unit. A systematic review yielded no apparent benefit of intermittent compression over compression stockings.[14]

Table 8-1
Indications, Contraindications, and Physiological Effects of Compression

Indications	Contraindications	Physiological Effects
Edema	CHF (uncontrolled)	Improves venous and lymphatic circulation
Residual limb formation	Advanced peripheral neuropathy	Controls shape and size of tissue
Control of scarring	Abscesses	Increases tissue temperature
Treatment/prevention of venous stasis ulcers	Advanced peripheral obstructive arterial disease	
Prevention of DVTs	DVT (once patient has been diagnosed with one)	

What the research does agree on, however, is that compression can do a very effective job of treating and preventing venous stasis ulcers.[15,16] The research does not show that compression garments or wraps do a better job than intermittent compression, but it does support any kind of compression over none at all. Venous stasis ulcers develop as a result of chronic edema, which in this case often results from a dysfunction of the valves in veins that usually keeps fluid from going back down into the extremities. Fluid collects in the lower extremities, and this increased pressure can cause ulcers to form. Often, venous stasis ulcers are noted on or around the ankle. Because the cause of these ulcers is the dysfunction of venous valves and the effects of gravity, compression can either help prevent new venous ulcers from forming or facilitate their healing. This makes patients who have venous stasis ulcers good candidates for compression.

The need for residual limb formation or scar healing and formation are additional indications for compression. As mentioned previously, a residual limb needs to be a specific shape to fit into a prosthetic socket. Individuals who are prone to hypertrophic or keloid scars can benefit from compression's effects.

Although compression can benefit a variety of patients, there are contraindications for its use. These include advanced peripheral neuropathy, which is when a patient lacks sensation in the peripheral limbs, abscesses, infection, CHF, and advanced peripheral obstructive arterial disease.[17] If the patient lacks sensation, they cannot accurately report sensation during the compression intervention, and you may inadvertently obstruct blood flow. Abscesses and infections, especially in the local area, can be transmitted to other areas of the body because compression increases circulation. If a patient has CHF, the heart is already unable to sufficiently pump fluid throughout the body; compression adds additional fluid and may overload the heart. Any obstruction of the lymphatic or venous/arterial system is problematic because an obstruction prevents fluid from moving appropriately and can back up at the blockage. In addition, it is worth noting that although compression is often used to prevent DVTs, it is not indicated to be used once a DVT has been diagnosed because it can dislodge the clot and cause further damage. While cancer is not usually listed as a contraindication, it can at least be considered a precaution because the increased circulation can, again, promote movement of cells from one area to another. A list of all indications, contraindications, and physiological effects of compression is provided in Table 8-1.

APPLICATION METHODS

It has already been mentioned that there are a variety of ways for compression to be applied to the body. The easiest and cheapest method to provide compression is with the use of elastic wraps. Some situations require the need for more advanced compression garments, which can be either off the shelf or custom made. Finally, intermittent pneumatic compression pumps are another compression option for patients. Each type of compression will be discussed at length.

Wraps

Compression wraps or bandages are relatively inexpensive and can be found easily. Figure 8-3 shows various wraps. They work either via resting or working pressure. Wraps that are more elastic work via resting pressure and are most often used with patients who are less mobile or bedridden. The elastic wraps exert pressure against the tissues whether the patient does or does not move. These wraps are also often referred to as *long-stretch* or *high-stretch bandages* (Figure 8-4) and are usually able to provide 60 to 70 mm Hg of pressure. Ace bandages are examples of long-stretch bandages, and they can create more pressure (measured in mm Hg). Less elastic or inelastic wraps, by comparison, produce a working pressure, which is when an active muscle presses against the inelastic bandage. These bandages are often called *short-stretch* or *low-stretch bandages* (Figure 8-5).

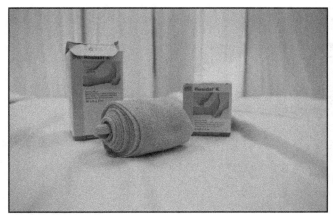

Figure 8-3. Variety of wraps.

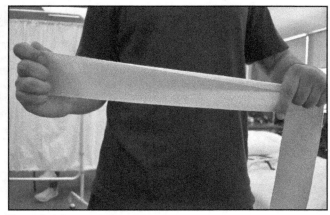

Figure 8-4. Long-stretch wraps.

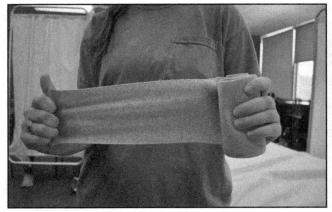

Figure 8-5. Short-stretch wraps.

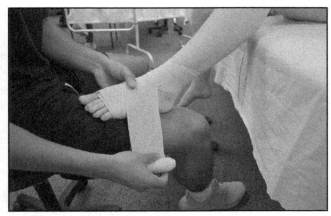

Figure 8-6. Figure-of-8 pattern.

Some patients receive multiple layers of wraps around an extremity. For example, when patients with lymphedema are wrapped, they receive a combination of cotton batting, long-stretch, and short-stretch bandages to manage the swelling. This wrapping follows a series of massage techniques to prime specific lymph nodes to accept the fluid and to move the fluid in that direction. Physical therapist assistants can obtain specific training and certification in the treatment of lymphedema, including what types of bandages to use, in what order, and in what form. The wrapping may be performed in the preferred figure-of-8 form (Figure 8-6) or a spiral form (Figure 8-7), but a circular method should be avoided to prevent a tourniquet effect.

To treat venous stasis ulcers, the patient will receive typical wound care interventions and the compression bandage will both protect the wound as well as provide compression to address venous insufficiency. An Unna boot, which is a bandage impregnated with zinc oxide, provides 35 to 40 mm Hg of pressure. They are soft on application but harden to make a semi-rigid boot. The patient wears this boot for up to a few weeks, when it is then removed and replaced.

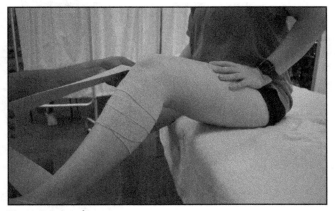

Figure 8-7. Spiral pattern.

Regardless of the type of wrap, a few general rules apply. Pressure should be greater distally and less as the wrap moves proximally. Typically, the wrap attempts to cover the entire limb (leaving no exposed areas of the limb). Also, there should be no wrinkles in the wrap to prevent uneven pressure and the potential to cause new or worsening wounds. Table 8-2 lists the details on how to apply compression wraps.

Table 8-2	
Procedures for Applying Compression Wraps	
Equipment Needed	• Wraps/bandages of varying stretch • Cotton or foam for padding or absorbency
Treatment/ Parameters	• Confirm patient does not have contraindications. • Determine optimal patient position—supine or short sit might be easiest. • Remove clothing and jewelry from area. • Dress any wounds, as needed. • Apply bandage, starting distally, with more compression, and work proximally. You may use the figure-of-8 or spiral wrap technique. You may find it easier to unroll the bandage from under rather than over. • When treatment is complete, assess patient's response.
Safety Considerations	• Monitor patient's response (verbally and visually) during treatment session; adjust treatment accordingly. • Check patient's sensation and look for good coloring of extremities.
Advantages	• Inexpensive • Easy to apply once skill is mastered • Easy to access wraps • Extremity can be used even after wraps are applied
Disadvantages	• Does not reverse edema • Requires moderate skill to apply correctly • Difficult to quantify compression • Bulky, hot, and unattractive

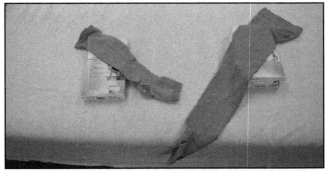

Figure 8-8. Compression garments.

Compression wraps can be difficult to apply to oneself, and some training is required to do it correctly. They can be bulky, hot, and some patients do not find them terribly attractive. While they are effective in reducing edema, they are not effective in reversing edema, and it is difficult to determine exactly how much pressure a wrap is exerting.

Garments

While wraps are easily accessible and relatively inexpensive, they may not provide the compression a patient requires. Compression garments can be "off the shelf," meaning they apply a certain specific amount of pressure (usually indicated on the box) and come in a variety of sizes, or they can be custom made per measurements taken of the patient's extremity.

Off-the-shelf garments include external compression stockings, or antiembolism stockings (sometimes referred to as *TED hose*). These are given to any patient in the hospital to help prevent DVTs. These have a low level of compression (16 to 18 mm Hg) and can be either knee high or thigh high. Patients are expected to wear the stockings all day, every day, until they are mobile enough to prevent DVTs through muscle movement. Other off-the-shelf garments include generic stockings used by patients going on long airplane rides or by pregnant individuals looking to decrease the swelling suffered during late pregnancy, and these provide 30 to 40 mm Hg of pressure. Figure 8-8 shows some examples of compression garments.

Custom-fit garments are usually commissioned for chronic or long-term concerns. Patients who have had an amputation and need their residual limb formed or shaped may need a custom garment to provide sufficient pressure. Patients who have had burns to their bodies or have extensive scarring will need garments measured to fit their

Table 8-3
Procedures for Applying Compression Garments

Equipment Needed	• Compression garment of appropriate compression amount
Treatment/ Parameters	• Confirm patient does not have contraindications. • Determine optimal patient position—supine or short sit might be easiest. • Remove clothing and jewelry from area. • Apply garment; educate patient or caregiver on application and fit of garment. • When treatment is complete, assess patient's response. • Compression garments for varicose veins: 20 to 30 mm Hg; compression garments for venous ulcers 30 to 40 mm Hg; compression for lymphedema 40 to 50 mm Hg; compression for mild venous insufficiency 10 to 20 mm Hg; compression for burns or scars: 20 to 30 mm Hg.
Safety Considerations	• Monitor patient's response (verbally and visually). • Check patient's sensation and look for good coloring of extremities. • Check fit of the garment to see if it needs to be replaced; garments should be replaced at least every 6 months, although more frequently if worn daily, such as with burns or chronic conditions.
Advantages	• Compression can be measured • Extremity can be used after garment is applied • Garments come in variety of colors and patterns, so are more attractive and less bulky • Less expensive than intermittent compression units • Can be worn 24 hours/day
Disadvantages	• Does not reverse edema • More expensive than compression wraps • Must be fitted appropriately • Can be hot • Requires some strength and dexterity to apply • Must be replaced at least every 6 mo and must have 2 garments (wash and wear)

bodies exactly; 20 to 30 mm Hg of pressure is recommended for scar tissue treatment. Patients with lymphedema will first undergo many repetitions of compression wrapping to shrink the extremity to a desired size; once that is accomplished and the limb size is stable, they will be fitted for a specific garment to help maintain the new size. Custom-fit garments will need to be replaced after a certain amount of use because the elastic will stretch out. Also, if the patient gains or loses weight, or if the extremity in question changes size, the custom garment should be replaced.

Compression garments can be difficult to don and doff, so patients and/or their caregivers will need to be trained. Patients should have at least 2 stockings (1 to wash and 1 to wear). They can be hot, but they do come in a variety of colors and patterns so patients find them more attractive than wraps. Like wraps, they cannot reverse edema, but they can help control edema, and unlike wraps, garments

can apply quantifiable compression. Table 8-3[18] discusses the application of compression garments and the pressure they provide.

Intermittent Compression

In the hospital, one may notice that patients in bed wear Velcro-closed compression devices on the lower extremities. These are connected via tubes to an electrical unit hanging from the base of the bed (Figure 8-9), and they inflate and deflate intermittently. These are one example of intermittent compression. Like wraps and garments, intermittent compression aims to prevent DVTs and reduce swelling; they differ in that they are able to provide segmental or sequential compression up a limb and they can both control and potentially reverse edema. Intermittent compression can be used in the hospital, in the therapy clinic, or at home. The sleeves can either be single chambered, which

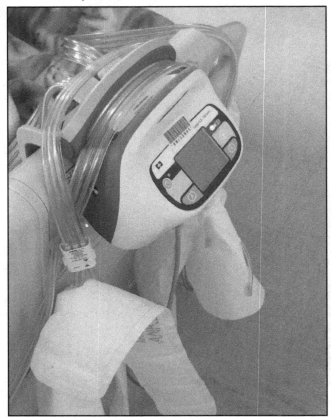

Figure 8-9. Intermittent compression in hospital setting.

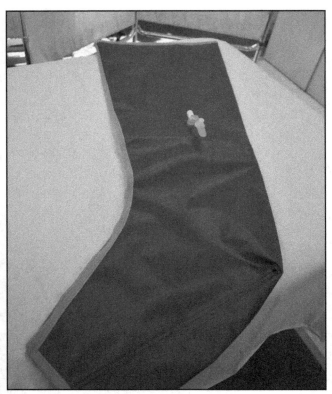

Figure 8-10. Single sleeve.

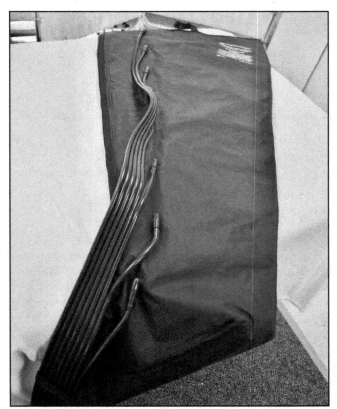

Figure 8-11. Multichamber sleeve.

inflate and deflate all at once, or they can have individual chambers that sequentially inflate and deflate up the limb. Figure 8-10 shows a single-chamber sleeve, and Figure 8-11 shows a multichamber sleeve. The latter can be advantageous because it mimics muscle contraction and the normal movement of fluid up a limb. Figure 8-12 shows a patient set-up with a compression sleeve. The patient must wear a stockinette (Figure 8-13) under the compression sleeve to control sweating and protect the skin.

While beneficial for edema or lymphedema, as well as for the prevention of DVTs, intermittent compression is not effective in preventing excessive scarring since it can be worn for only a few hours at a time. Also, the patient is unable to get up and move around while wearing the unit. Intermittent compression may work even better if the limb being treated is in an elevated position. Figures 8-14 and 8-15 show older and newer models of intermittent compression units.

While there are no agreed-on parameters for intermittent compression, the general consensus is that the maximum compression to a limb should not exceed a patient's diastolic blood pressure number or 60 mm Hg for the upper extremity and 80 mm Hg for the lower extremity (whichever is lower). However, a systematic review of the use of intermittent pneumatic compression demonstrates the varied compression dosage. The review says that compressions of 5 to 10 mm Hg to greater than 120 mm Hg were effective in the studies, but that average peak inflations of 25 to

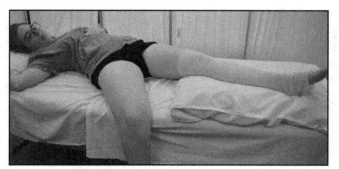

Figure 8-12. Stockinette on patient.

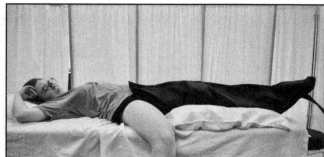

Figure 8-13. Patient positioning with sleeve.

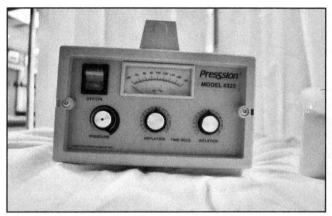

Figure 8-14. Older intermittent compression pump.

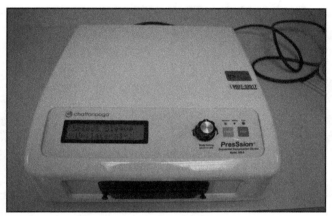

Figure 8-15. Newer intermittent compression pump.

50 mm Hg were sufficient for most patients.[19] Intermittent compression units vary in their complexity, often correlated to whether the sleeve is multichambered or single chambered, but almost all allow for customization of on/off time (usually a 3:1 ratio), the pressure, and the total time of the treatment. Table 8-4 details the application of intermittent compression.

As with many modalities, intermittent compression can be combined with other modalities. Compression and ice, for example, are common combinations to reduce swelling. The cryocuff system, as mentioned in a previous chapter, is an example of cold and compression being used in combination to reduce both pain and swelling. A future chapter will discuss electrical stimulation and how it can, among other things, reduce swelling. A therapist could apply electrodes and administer electrical stimulation in combination with compression to reduce swelling. The next chapter discusses soft-tissue mobilization or massage, which is also often combined with compression to promote the removal of excess fluid in tissues. The use of massage is a key component in the treatment of lymphedema.

SAFETY CONCERNS

As with all modalities, compression requires the therapist to monitor the patient's response to the treatment. This may be a verbal response, but often the patient's response may come in the form of facial expressions or body language. While compression can be uncomfortable, the patient should not experience significant pain or discomfort during the treatment. Check the patient's sensation and coloration in the distal portion of the extremity being treated to determine that nerve function and blood flow has not been occluded or damaged. In cases of intermittent compression, monitor the patient's blood pressure during the treatment to make sure it is neither dropping nor elevating in response to the treatment. If the patient complains of dizziness, lightheadedness, or nausea or shows other physical signs of blood pressure changes, stop the treatment.

When applying wraps or garments, the therapist should take care to avoid wrinkles or gaps and to check the patient's skin after removing the wraps or garments to ensure the patient's skin is intact and healthy. For intermittent compression, a stockinette must be used to protect the patient's skin.

Table 8-4	
Procedures for Applying Intermittent Compression	
Equipment Needed	• Intermittent compression unit • Stockinette • Blood pressure cuff • Stethoscope • Tape measure • Pillows/sheets as needed
Treatment/ Parameters	• Confirm patient does not have contraindications. • Determine optimal patient position—supine or sitting might be easiest with extremity elevated if possible. • Remove clothing and jewelry from area. • Take patient's blood pressure. • Measure and record patient's circumferential girth at a variety of locations on the limb. • Apply stockinette and then apply compression sleeve. • Connect sleeve via hose to compression unit. • Select compression parameters; inflation should ≤ 60 mm Hg for the upper extremity or 80 mm Hg for the lower extremity, or ≤ patient's diastolic blood pressure number (whichever is lower); inflation/deflation time is a 3:1 ratio for total of 1 to 4 hours; frequency varies depending on indication and response to treatment. • Provide patient a call bell. • Remeasure limb after treatment is concluded. • Inspect patient's skin. • Apply a compression garment to help maintain reduction in swelling.
Safety Considerations	• Monitor patient's response (verbally and visually). • Check patient's sensation and look for good coloring of extremities. • If patient complains of feeling dizzy, lightheaded, or of pain during treatment, end treatment session.
Advantages	• Compression can be quantified • Can both reverse and control edema • Less complex to apply than bandages or garments • Can provide sequential compression if unit allows
Disadvantages	• Can be used for only a few hours at a time, so cannot control scarring • More expensive than wraps or garments; patient may have to come to therapy clinic for treatment • Requires use of electricity • Patient cannot move or use extremity during treatment session • Not indicated for acute injuries/conditions

DOCUMENTATION

Documentation of compression requires first noting the type of compression applied. Specify what part of the body is being treated and for what purpose. Indicate the position of the patient during the treatment. If wrapping the patient, indicate the type of wraps (short or long stretch), the pattern of wrapping used, and how many layers applied. If applying a garment, designate whether the garment is custom or off the shelf. If using intermittent compression, include the inflation/deflation times, the inflation pressure, and the total treatment time. Always include the patient's response to the treatment, and also include measurements of girth to show progress or change. See the following examples of documentation.

Diagnosis: Patient is in therapy because of having a right transtibial amputation status post 6 weeks ago. The patient's incision is healed, and he is now undergoing residual limb formation so he can wear a prosthetic and begin gait training.

O: Patient received compression wrapping to right residual limb for prosthetic preparation. Anchored wrap around right knee and used figure-of-8 form to wrap limb with pressure distal greater than proximal. Confirmed with patient intact sensation after wraps applied. Patient had no pain after treatment completed.

Diagnosis: Patient is in therapy to receive intermittent compression because of lymphedema following left breast mastectomy with lymph node removal.

O: Patient's blood pressure taken in the right upper extremity was 138/78 mm Hg. Applied stockinette to upper extremity and then sleeve; upper extremity elevated on wedge. Inflation/deflation set at 60 seconds and 20 seconds at 55 mm Hg × 60 minutes. Blood pressure was at 140/79 mm Hg and 136/78 mm Hg during the session.

Conclusion

Compression is a modality with which many are familiar, especially within the context of postacute injury treatment. There are a variety of compression options, ranging from the relatively inexpensive but difficult to apply wraps to the more expensive but more effective intermittent compression units. What one uses with patients will depend on the patient's diagnosis, progress with other treatments, and availability in the clinic. Compression can be combined with other modalities such as ice, electricity, and exercise to increase its effectiveness.

Review Questions

1. List the 3 types of compression and offer a brief description of each.
2. Define lymphedema. How does it differ from edema that results from a sprained ankle?
3. List and explain the physiological effects of compression.
4. What are the benefits of using compression wraps? Disadvantages?
5. List the parameters for intermittent compression.
6. What modalities can be used in combination with compression? How are they beneficial?
7. What are the contraindications for compression?

8. You are seeing a patient after an acutely sprained right wrist. The patient reports increased swelling by the end of the day. The patient is able to move the extremity but complains of 6/10 pain with movement. What type of compression intervention would you recommend? Why? Document your imaginary treatment session.

9. Your patient has a venous stasis ulcer on the medial malleolus of the left lower extremity, with measurements of 3 cm × 4 cm (no depth) and significant serosanguinous exudate. Girth measured at the left ankle is 11 inches; dorsiflexion is 0 to 15 degrees and plantar flexion is 0 to 20 degrees. What type of compression would you recommend and why? Document your treatment session.

Case Study 1

After sliding into second base during an amateur softball game, your 38-year-old patient has been referred to therapy with a left lateral ankle sprain. He initially followed instructions to elevate and ice the ankle, but now 72 hours later, he has stopped following those instructions and presents with a significantly swollen ankle. He can bear weight on the limb, but it is painful, 5/10 pain, and palpation is tender. He has reduced ROM as well. The goal is to reduce swelling to restore normal ROM and function and reduce pain.

1. What tissues are injured?
2. What phase of healing is the patient in?
3. What compression intervention would you recommend? Why?
4. What are the contraindications for this intervention?
5. Describe the parameters for this intervention.
6. What other modality (noncompression) would you recommend? Why?

Case Study 2

Your patient is a 44-year-old woman with chronic lymphedema in her right upper extremity after having a radical mastectomy because of a breast cancer diagnosis. Pain with swelling increases to 8/10, and she reports the limb feels heavy and is difficult to move through the full range in any direction. She finds it difficult to dress, and she would like to return to her work as an administrative assistant for the local college. Your instructions are to reduce the swelling to improve function and reduce pain.

1. What tissues are affected?
2. What compression intervention would you recommend? Why?
3. What parameters would you select for this intervention?
4. What is the difference between lymphedema and swelling associated with a musculoskeletal injury?

REFERENCES

1. Keast D. The science of compression. Lymphedemapathways.ca. Published 2012. Accessed April 12, 2020. https://canadalymph.ca/wp-content/uploads/2015/04/The-Science-of-Compression.pdf

2. Bayat A, McGrouther DA, Ferguson MW. Skin scarring. *BMJ*. 2003;326(7380):88-92.

3. Alkhalil A, Carney BC, Travis TE, et al. Key cell functions are modulated by compression in an animal model of hypertrophic scar. *Wounds*. 2018;30(12):353-362.

4. Juzo. Scar therapy: information and tips bout skin and scars. Accessed April 12, 2020. https://www.juzo.com/en/service-knowledge/well-informed/scar-therapy

5. Bleasdale B, Finnegan S, Murray K, Kelly S, Percival SL. The use of silicone adhesives for scar reduction. *Adv Wound Care (New Rochelle)*. 2015;4(7):422-430.

6. Sanders JE, Fatone S. Residual limb volume change: systematic review of measurement and management. *J Rehabil Res Dev*. 2011;48(8):949-986.

7. Mayo Clinic. Phantom pain. Published 2020. Accessed April 12, 2020. https://www.mayoclinic.org/diseases-conditions/phantom-pain/symptoms-causes/syc-20376272

8. NHS Inform. Amputation. Published 2020. Accessed April 12, 2020. https://www.nhsinform.scot/tests-and-treatments/surgical-procedures/amputation

9. Mayo Clinic. Lymphedema. Published 2017. Accessed April 19, 2020. https://www.mayoclinic.org/diseases-conditions/lymphedema/symptoms-causes/syc-20374682

10. Clarke M, Broderick C, Hopewell S, Juszczak E, Eisinga A. Compression stockings for preventing deep vein thrombosis in airline passengers. *Cochrane Database Syst Rev*. 2016;9(9):CD004002.

11. Naccarato M, Chiodo Grandi F, Dennis M, Sandercock PA. Physical methods for preventing deep vein thrombosis in stroke. *Cochrane Database Syst Rev*. 2010;(8):CD001922.

12. Kahn SR, Shapiro S, Wells PS, et al; SOX Trial Investigators. Compression stockings to prevent post-thrombotic syndrome: a randomised placebo-controlled trial. *Lancet*. 2014;383(9920):880-888.

13. CLOTS (Clots in Legs Or sTockings after Stroke) Trial Collaboration. Thigh-length versus below-knee stockings for deep venous thrombosis prophylaxis after stroke: a randomized trial. *Ann Intern Med*. 2010;153(9):553-562.

14. Morris RJ. Woodcock JP. Intermittent pneumatic compression or graduated compression stockings for deep vein thrombosis prophylaxis? A systematic review of direct clinical comparisons. *Ann Surg*. 2010;251(3):393-396.

15. Haesler E. Evidence summary: venous leg ulcers—pneumatic compression. *Wound Practice & Research*. 2019;27(3):147-148.

16. Rabe E, Rartsch H, Hafner J, et al. Indications for medical compression stockings in venous and lymphatic disorders: an evidence-based consensus statement. *Phlebology*. 2018;33(3):163-184.

17. Nair B. Compression therapy for venous leg ulcers. *Indian Dermatol Online J*. 2014;5(3):378-382.

18. Xiong Y, Tao X. Compression garments for medical therapy and sports. *Polymers (Basel)*. 2018;10(6):663.

19. Feldman JL, Stout NL, Wanchai BR, et al. Intermittent pneumatic compression therapy: a systematic review. *Lymphology*. 2012;45:13-25.

Chapter 9

Manual Therapy and Soft-Tissue Mobilization

KEY TERMS Effleurage | Fascia | Friction massage | Mechanical effects | Myofascial release | Petrissage | Reflexive effects | Tapotement | Trigger points | Vibration

KEY ABBREVIATION IASTM

CHAPTER OBJECTIVES

1. Describe what manual therapy and soft-tissue mobilization are and the different techniques of each.
2. Discuss the physiological effects of manual therapy and soft-tissue mobilization.
3. Discuss the guidelines and considerations for the application of manual therapy and soft-tissue mobilization as physical therapy interventions.
4. Explain the indications and contraindications for manual therapy and soft-tissue mobilization interventions.
5. Apply knowledge of manual therapy and soft-tissue mobilization set-up and parameters to case scenarios.
6. Document manual therapy and soft-tissue mobilization interventions correctly in a patient's chart.

INTRODUCTION

Manual therapy, or any kind of mechanical stimulation or manipulation of the tissues or joints, has been used for years to provide pain relief and promote flexibility and restore mobility. While this chapter will focus heavily on the basic techniques of soft-tissue mobilization (STM), or massage, it will also address other tissue mobilization techniques such as friction massage, myofascial release, and joint mobilization. A physical therapist assistant can become specially trained in certain mobilization techniques either formally or informally to work in coordination with other interventions to yield the desired patient outcome.

PHYSIOLOGICAL EFFECTS OF MANUAL THERAPY AND SOFT-TISSUE MOBILIZATION

Manual therapy and STM typically yield either a reflexive or mechanical effect on the tissue. Sometimes, one might also consider the psychological effects of these methods.

Reflexive Effects

Perhaps the most obvious effects of any manual therapy are those on the sensory receptors of the skin and superficial connective tissues. When hands glide lightly over the tissues, the sensory receptors are stimulated and the recipient may feel relaxed and a reduction of pain. Reflexive effects also include those on circulation and possibly metabolism.

Pain

Specifically, STM is argued to decrease pain, likely via the Gate Control theory, as superficial sensory nerves (Aβ fibers) are stimulated, blocking out the slower Aδ or C pain fibers. In cases of more aggressive mobilization, the Opiate theory may also be a cause for pain reduction when painful areas are stimulated during mobilization. Either way, many

99

Box 9-1

Research Topic

Create a patient, intervention, comparison, outcome, time question to address the use of STM techniques to treat tendinopathy. What research exists on this topic, and what does it have to say? Is it conclusive? What STM techniques are recommended, based on the current research? Do any of the studies compare the use of STM to other modality interventions, and if so, what are the outcomes?

studies support the concept that pain can be reduced and relaxation promoted via STM techniques,[1,2] although these same studies vary on how significant the pain reduction is or how long the pain reduction lasts.

Circulation

In addition to pain reduction, STM can affect circulation.[3] When a person receives a massage, is it not uncommon to notice that the treatment area becomes flushed or darker/pinker as blood flow is affected. Superficial blood vessels are affected by the light touch of reflexive massage techniques. Additionally, massage can increase tissue temperature, which, in turn, can cause vasodilation and increase circulation.[4]

In addition to increasing circulation, massage can influence lymphatic fluid flow. When applying certain types of massage to an area, one might note that swelling in the area is also decreased (eg, massage is a significant component of lymphedema treatment). In the previous chapter, compression was discussed as an effective method to reduce or even reverse edema. Often, compression is used in tandem with massage to further reduce or control edema.

Metabolism and Immunity

While there is no evidence that massage directly influences metabolism, some research indicates that massage can decrease the incidence or severity of delayed-onset muscle soreness (DOMS).[5,6] In addition to decreasing pain after exercise, massage has known relaxation effects on the body. There has been new research studying the effects of stress on the human body, especially the immune response as it correlates to stress.[7] In studies with babies,[8] mice,[9] and adults,[10] massage has been shown to increase T and B lymphocyte activity, thus boosting the immune system. More research is needed in both of these areas to support the veracity of these claims.

Mechanical Effects

While reflexive effects are correlated to superficial techniques that glide over the skin, mechanical effects involve manual manipulation, stretching, or mobilization of the muscles, tendons, or skin. Mechanical techniques, then, address deeper as well as superficial tissues.

Muscle and Tendon

The effects of STM on DOMS were previously discussed. Deeper effects on muscle tissue include increasing the length of muscles, although massage has no effect on muscle strength.[11] Massage may also improve muscle healing after an injury by increasing angiogenesis, decreasing muscle fibrosis, and stimulating endogenous muscle stem cells to secrete vascular endothelial growth factor.[12] Mechanical techniques can reduce the pain noted in myofascial trigger points.[13] Trigger points, a symptom or component of myofascial pain syndrome, often result from repetitive actions or postures, yield tenderness and referred pain,[14] and can result in limited range of motion (ROM) or headaches. Massage techniques can release the tension in the tissue as well as the underlying fascia, decreasing pain and improving mobility. Tendon pain may be addressed with deeper massage techniques, and it is common for therapists to employ cross-friction massage to decrease sensitivity in tendinopathy or tendinitis cases. Box 9-1 suggests a research topic on the use of STM for the treatment of tendinopathy. Additionally, some studies are showing that massage coupled with physical activity can aid in tendon repair by stimulating fibroblast metabolic activity and causing the fibroblasts to secrete transforming growth factor β, prostaglandin E2, and leukotriene B4.[15]

Skin

As mentioned previously, massage can increase superficial tissue temperature. Massage is also often used to decrease the severity and limitations of scar tissue. As mentioned in the Compression chapter (Chapter 8), scar tissue can limit ROM and function; some scars, such as keloid or hypertrophic, can yield even worse outcomes. While scarring is a normal process of healing, some scars adhere to the tissues below and restrict motion. The application of massage to scar tissue can increase the flexibility of the scar and reduce pain associated with it, as well as improve ROM.[16]

Psychological Effects

Massage can have relaxing effects on the recipient, especially effleurage and certain petrissage techniques. Some studies have shown that massage can reduce both psychological and physical distress,[17] while others show that massage can produce comfort, reduce anxiety, and improve the quality of sleep in acute and critical care patients.[18,19] It is thought that stress increases the levels of cortisol released by the hypothalamus, and that even one massage treatment can reduce cortisol levels for 30 to 120 minutes after the treatment.[20] These psychological benefits can be just as influential in patient outcomes as the reflexive and mechanical effects.

Table 9-1
Indications, Contraindications, and Physiological Effects of Soft-Tissue Mobilization/Massage

Indications	Contraindications	Physiological Effects
Edema	Over open wounds	Improves venous and lymphatic circulation
Decreased ROM	Over rashes	Decreases pain via Gate Control theory or Opiate theory
Decreased joint mobility	Over abscesses	Decrease size/severity of scar tissue
DOMS	Over infections	Reduce myofascial trigger points
Scar tissue	Deep vein thrombosis (once patient has been diagnosed with one)	Promote tendon healing
Trigger points	Cancer	Increase immune response
Muscle spasms	Over insertion sites of intravenous lines, tubes, shunts, etc	Promote relaxation, decrease cortisol levels, promote improved sleep
Tendinitis	Over acute fractures	

INDICATIONS AND CONTRAINDICATIONS OF MANUAL THERAPY AND SOFT-TISSUE MOBILIZATION

It makes sense when looking at the aforementioned effects of massage that indications for massage include just about anything that involves muscles, connective tissue, tendons, and joints. These include muscle spasms, trigger points, adhesions, edema, decreased ROM, tendinopathy, bursitis, DOMS, scar tissue, decreased joint mobility, and, of course, pain of any sort.

Contraindications for massage include performing massage over or around open wounds, including areas of tissue showing erythema. One should avoid massage over rashes, infections, or cellulitis.[20] Intravenous insertion sites, incisions, acute fractures, or drains, shunts, and other tubes are also contraindicated areas for massage.[20] If a patient has a known deep vein thrombosis or thrombosis, massage should be avoided until the patient is cleared. If a patient has known cancer in the area, massage may be contraindicated; one does not want to cause metastasis, which is possible due to the increased circulation caused by massage; however, in some cases, massage might be a pain-relieving technique. Table 9-1 lists the indications, contraindications, and physiological effects of STM.

APPLICATION OF METHODS

There are a variety of massage or STM techniques one can use with a patient, and this text cannot discuss all of

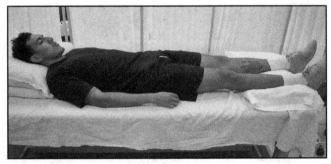

Figure 9-1. Supine position of comfort.

the possible methods. However, we will focus on some of the most common techniques used in the clinic. Bear in mind that some of these methods might require additional continuing education or certification.

Technique Guidelines

Massage and STM comes with their own guidelines and considerations to ensure the techniques are administered correctly. In addition to knowing basic anatomy and physiology, the physical therapist assistant should make sure the patient is positioned and draped properly to provide warmth, to protect the patient's clothing, to prevent pressure build-up, to access the body part(s) required, and to provide modesty for the patient. Positions of comfort are the ideal: in supine, have a pillow under the head and knees; in prone, have a pillow under the abdomen or lower extremities. Figures 9-1 and 9-2 show positions of comfort in supine and prone. If the patient is sitting (Figure 9-3),

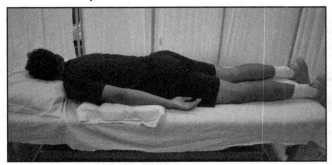

Figure 9-2. Prone position of comfort.

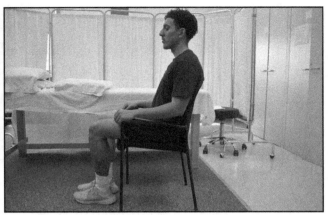

Figure 9-3. Sitting position for massage.

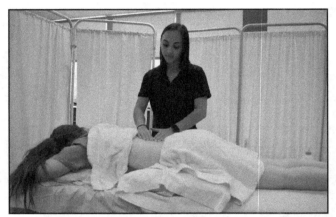

Figure 9-4. Therapist applying massage while standing with proper body mechanics.

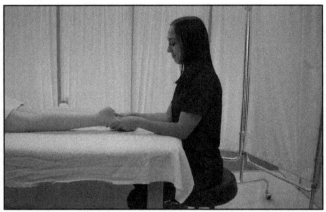

Figure 9-5. Therapist sitting to apply massage.

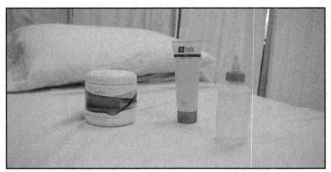

Figure 9-6. Baby oil and cocoa butter.

they should be positioned in neutral. Another option could have the patient leaning forward on a table with a pillow for support. The patient's comfort should be established before the treatment session.

The therapist's nails should be clean and short so as not to scratch the patient. The therapist should wash their hands and make sure hands are warm before touching the patient. The therapist should always explain to the patient in advance what will happen during the treatment session; this is especially important if the therapist is going to be touching around or near sensitive areas of the body. The therapist should maintain proper body mechanics, meaning that the treatment table is raised or lowered, if possible,

so the therapist can reach the patient and distribute weight evenly on both feet. The therapist may need a step stool or to sit down to maintain body mechanics. Figures 9-4 and 9-5 show a therapist adhering to proper body mechanics.

A small amount of lubricant is all that is needed for most massage techniques. There are some methods that do not call for lubricant. There are a variety of lubricants one can use for massage; baby oil or cocoa butter are common lubricants. Figure 9-6 shows some common lubricants used in massage. Ensure the patient is not allergic to the lubricant used. Typically, a small amount of rubbing alcohol on a towel can be used to remove the lubricant once the session is completed.

Once contact is made with the patient's body, it is ideal to not break contact; if the therapist needs to move to another side of the body, keep one hand on the patient while moving. This helps keep the patient relaxed. Also avoid talking too much during the session. It is okay to ask about pressure or comfort, but do not have a conversation during the session. The amount of pressure used depends on the treatment purpose and the patient response. Some patients like more or less pressure, and some interventions, such as myofascial release, require more pressure to accomplish the

Table 9-2
General Techniques for Massage
Position and drape patient for warmth, modesty, comfort, protection of clothing, and access to body part.
Therapist's nails should be clean and trimmed.
Educate/communicate with patient before treatment.
Maintain proper body mechanics.
Use a small amount of lubricant on hands first (not poured on patient).
Do not break contact with patient's body after beginning session.
Avoid excessive talking.
Check on patient response to pressure and adjust accordingly.
Move from proximal to distal if addressing edema.
Begin and end session with effleurage.

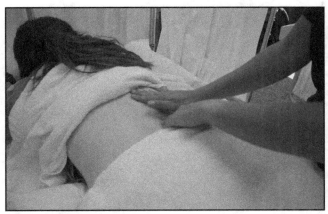

Figure 9-7. Massage in direction of muscle fibers.

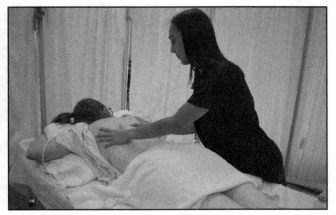

Figure 9-8. Effleurage stroke.

goal. The therapist should listen to the patient's feedback and make adjustments accordingly.

Use the entire hand, not just the fingertips or heel of the hand, and use a steady, regular rhythm. Typically, one will follow the direction of the muscle fibers (Figure 9-7). If one is massaging to help with edema, move from distal to proximal, unless applying lymphedema massage, in which case one starts proximally to facilitate lymphatic flow, and then moves from distal to proximal. If possible, elevate the body part being treated.

One should aim to begin and end a massage session with effleurage; this technique is relaxing, allows the patient to become accustomed to the therapist's touch, moves the lubricant over the tissue, and reduces pain. Use a light touch over bony prominences and joints. Table 9-2 provides this list of general massage to-dos.

Soft-Tissue Mobilization/Massage

When thinking of "classic" massage, which includes effleurage, petrissage, tapotement, and vibration, one is thinking of what Albert Hoffa wrote about in *Technik der*

Massage, first published in 1893.[21] Each technique will be discussed here in a little more detail.

Effleurage

Effleurage is a light, gliding stroke that should be used to begin and end a massage session, as well as between other techniques used. It allows the patient to become accustomed to the therapist's touch, while also spreading the lubricant over the tissue and initiation some circulatory effects on the tissue. It also allows the therapist to get a "feel" for the patient's tissues and search out areas they may want to address later in the session, such as trigger points or muscle spasms. The therapist should use their full hand and follow the muscle fibers and should move toward the heart. Figure 9-8 shows a basic effleurage technique.

Petrissage

Petrissage, while still a relatively light touch, involves the picking up and kneading of tissues. The muscle and tissues are lifted and rolled or pressed under the fingers and

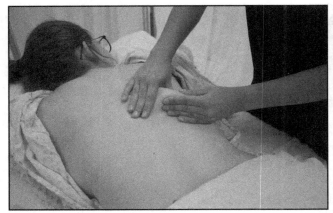

Figure 9-9. Kneading.

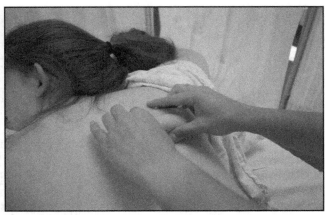

Figure 9-10. Rolling.

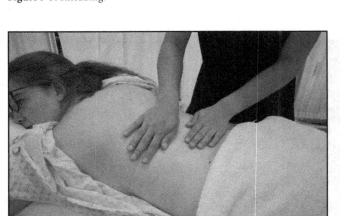

Figure 9-11. Parallel stroking.

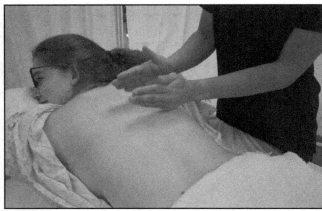

Figure 9-12. Hacking.

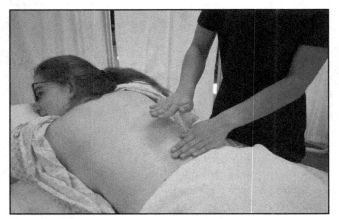

Figure 9-13. Slapping.

Tapotement

Tapotement is another word for percussion, and it involves brisk blows from relaxed hands in alternating movements. The names of the techniques sound a bit violent: hacking, slapping, beating, cupping. However, the words "relaxed hands" are important to remember during these treatments. Tapotement increases local circulation and stimulates peripheral nerve endings. Hacking is like a "karate chop": strike the patient with the ulnar side of the hand with relaxed wrists and hands (Figure 9-12). Slapping is using the whole fingers to alternately strike the patient's tissues (Figure 9-13). Beating uses a half-closed fist (like a "C" shape) and again striking on the ulnar side of the therapist's hands (Figure 9-14). Cupping, which is often used as a means to promote respiratory drainage and can be coupled with postural drainage techniques, involves making a concave surface with the hands and alternately clapping against the tissue. Figure 9-15 shows cupping.

hands; gliding only occurs to move the therapist's hands from one location to another. These techniques move fluid toward the heart and can help break up adhesions or begin to work on trigger points as well as relax muscle spasms. Kneading is one type of petrissage (Figure 9-9); other techniques include rolling and parallel stroking (Figures 9-10 and 9-11).

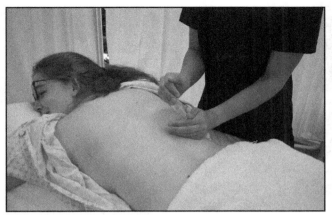

Figure 9-14. Beating.

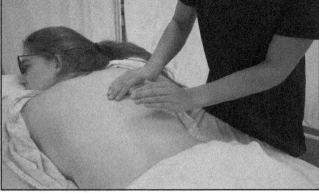

Figure 9-15. Cupping.

Vibration

As mentioned previously, cupping is commonly used as part of a postural drainage technique. Patients with upper respiratory infections or patients with cystic fibrosis are good candidates for cupping. Vibration is also used to help with respiratory drainage. The therapist places their hands firmly over the treatment area and then provides fine vibratory movements using the whole forearm (Figure 9-16). Table 9-3 provides the specifics on the application of STM or massage.

Friction Massage

Friction massage is a technique used and promoted by James Cyriax and Gillean Russell, and its purpose is to address pain or dysfunction in deeper structures such as tendons, ligaments, and deep muscles.[22] In the previous section, recommendations for massage included following along with the muscle fibers; friction massage desires movement perpendicular to or against the fibers. Friction massage requires the therapist to be well familiar with anatomical structures and to be able to palpate where the massage should occur. In addition, friction massage addresses a small surface area, unlike the previously discussed massage techniques that can cover a large area of the body. The pressure should be deep enough to move the skin and the structures beneath without causing blistering or other damage to the skin.

Friction massage hopes to accomplish 2 goals: to align and lengthen tissue fibers as they heal and to cause traumatic hyperemia to increase blood supply to the injured area.[22] Doing this enhances the natural inflammatory response to injury and allows the tissue to move through the latter phases of healing to return function and decrease pain.[22]

Friction massage requires the therapist to use the fingertips, thumbs, or heel of the hand to supply sufficient pressure to the area. Typically, the treatment is performed for trigger points or over nonacutely painful tendons/

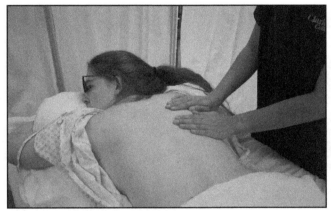

Figure 9-16. Vibration.

ligaments. A trigger point can be identified as a small nodule or lump in the muscle; sometimes when it is palpated, it feels grainy. On palpation, the patient may wince or withdraw in pain, and sometimes pain can radiate to another area of the body. Although initial treatment may be uncomfortable, some patients say it is the kind of pain that "hurts so good" in that it relieves pain in the long run. The therapist can apply deep pressure to the trigger point and then make small circular motions over the localized point. Figure 9-17 shows a friction massage treatment. Alternately, the therapist can perform a transverse movement perpendicular to the tissue fibers, such as in the case with tendinopathy (Figure 9-18).

When treating a tendon, it is best to put the tendon on a slight stretch and then use the thumb or fingers (overlapped if necessary) to create intense pressure while massaging the area. This is uncomfortable, to say the least, so patient education is important. Whereas massage can reduce pain via the Gate Control theory, friction massage works more via the Opiate theory, in that the noxious stimulus causes the release of natural endorphins in the body. Table 9-4 details the specifics on how to apply friction massage.

	Table 9-3
	Procedures for Applying Soft-Tissue Mobilization/Massage
Equipment Needed	• Lubricant • Towels, sheets, pillows • Treatment table/chair • Timer
Treatment/ Parameters	• Confirm patient does not have contraindications. • Educate patient on techniques being used and gain consent. • Determine optimal patient position—supine, prone, or seated. • Remove clothing and jewelry from area. • Apply lubricant on your hands and warm up before touching patient; make sure it is enough to glide over tissues without preventing deeper techniques. • Apply massage techniques. Begin with effleurage that progressively gets deeper. Work on petrissage and tapotement. Finish with deeper effleurage progressing to lighter strokes at the end. • Duration is variable; a larger area may require up to 30 min of massage; a localized treatment area may need only 10 min. • Ask patient for feedback on pressure and comfort and adjust treatment accordingly. • Use rubbing alcohol on a towel to clean off area after treatment. • Check with patient after treatment.
Safety Considerations	• Monitor patient's response (verbally and visually) during treatment session; adjust pressure accordingly. • Follow along muscle fibers and use caution over bony prominences. • Therapist should adhere to proper body mechanics during treatment.
Advantages	• Inexpensive • Easy to apply once skill is mastered • Can reduce edema in an area • Can reduce pain so patient can perform other activities
Disadvantages	• Patient is unable to use extremity/body or perform activities during treatment • May not have long-term effects on pain or muscle length • Does not strengthen muscles

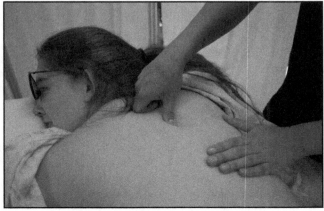

Figure 9-17. Friction massage (circular).

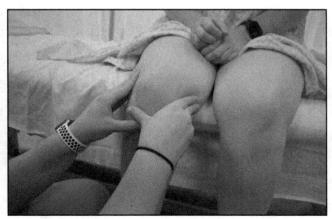

Figure 9-18. Transverse massage over tendon.

Table 9-4

Procedures for Applying Friction Massage

Equipment Needed	• Sheets, pillows • Treatment table/chair • Timer
Treatment/ Parameters	• Confirm patient does not have contraindications. • Determine optimal patient position—supine, prone, or seated. • Remove clothing and jewelry from area. • Confirm that patient understands friction massage will be uncomfortable but helpful. • No lubricant is used with friction massage. • Apply massage techniques. • Duration is variable, but usually ≤ 10 to 15 min because of intensity of treatment and small treatment area. • Check with patient after treatment; can apply ice to area before and after massage to help with discomfort.
Safety Considerations	• Monitor patient's response (verbally and visually) during treatment session. • Go against muscle fibers; make sure skin is moving with underlying tissues to avoid injury. • Therapist should adhere to proper body mechanics during treatment.
Advantages	• Inexpensive • Easy to apply once skill is mastered
Disadvantages	• Patient is unable to use extremity/body or perform activities during treatment • Treatment is uncomfortable so patient must be educated on its benefits

Myofascial Techniques

Myofascial techniques, sometimes called *myofascial release*, can address trigger points as discussed previously or can generally provide release of tight fascia combining pressure and stretch. The idea is that the fascia adheres to the skin above and the other structures below, limiting mobility and causing dysfunction and pain. As with friction massage, myofascial techniques typically do not use any lubricant and the treatment itself can, at times, be uncomfortable. Often, therapists well versed in myofascial techniques will perform an overall assessment of the patient to determine areas of tightness, rotation, or ROM limitations.

Myofascial release for trigger points is similar to that of friction massage; intense pressure is placed over the trigger point and held for a period of time (usually 1 to 5 minutes). The therapist can use fingers, thumbs, or even elbows to apply the pressure. The therapist can feel the trigger point release or relax under the fingers during the treatment, although one session is usually not enough to fully address the issue.

Myofascial release for other tissues involves the stretching of deeper tissues, including the fascia, with a low-load, long-duration method.[23] The goal is to decrease pain and increase function or mobility. As with trigger point therapy, significant pressure is required to reach the underlying tissues and fascia. Table 9-5 discusses how to apply myofascial techniques. There are a variety of techniques one can use, but a few include the cross-hands technique, the J-stroke, and skin rolling. One can become certified or specifically trained in myofascial techniques, in which many other skills can be learned and practiced.

Cross-hands (Figure 9-19) requires the therapist to place one hand on one side of the treatment area, then the other hand on the other side, so that the hands (and upper extremities) are crossed. The therapist then leans in and applies deep pressure while letting the hands slide out in opposite directions; this stretches the tissue in addition to the pressure provided. The idea is to hold this for at least 90 seconds, and as the hands move, feel where the movement stops. This may indicate a restriction, and the hands can be lifted and replaced over this new area to perform the technique again.

The J-stroke involves the therapist making a J-shape in the tissue; using the finger pads of 2 or 3 fingers, apply pressure over an area of restriction and move the fingers in the shape of a J. Apply this until the restriction feels released. See Figure 9-20 as an example.

Table 9-5	
Procedures for Applying Myofascial Techniques	
Equipment Needed	• Sheets, pillows • Treatment table/chair • Timer
Treatment/ Parameters	• Confirm patient does not have contraindications. • Determine optimal patient position—supine, prone, or seated. • Remove clothing and jewelry from area. • Apply massage techniques. Myofascial release for trigger points requires application of pressure using fingers, thumbs, or elbow over trigger point to decrease pain. Myofascial release elsewhere involves applying deep pressure to an area and a prolonged stretch. Some techniques include cross-hands, J-stroke, and skin rolling. • Duration is variable; 1 to 5 min is appropriate for trigger points; ≤ 10 min may be appropriate for other locations. • Check with patient after treatment.
Safety Considerations	• Monitor patient's response (verbally and visually) during treatment session. • Ensure skin and underlying tissues are moving so there is no damage to superficial tissues. • Therapist should adhere to proper body mechanics during treatment.
Advantages	• Inexpensive • Easy to apply once skill is mastered • Can reduce pain so patient can perform other activities
Disadvantages	• Patient is unable to use extremity/body or perform activities during treatment • Pain relief may not result from one treatment session

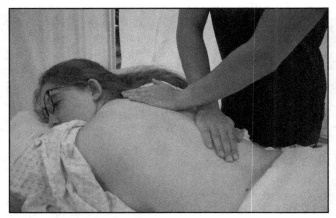

Figure 9-19. Cross-hands technique.

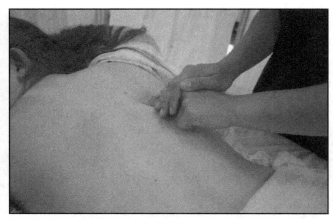

Figure 9-20. J-stroke.

Similar to petrissage, in that tissue is picked up and mobilized, skin rolling involves the therapist picking up a roll of skin and then using the thumbs and fingers to "walk" the skin roll up or across the tissues. You will feel that certain areas are easier to roll than others; those areas less easy to roll may indicate locations of adhesions and may benefit from other massage techniques.

Instrument-Assisted Soft-Tissue Mobilization

There are several different brand-name examples of instrument-assisted STM (IASTM) techniques, such as Graston and HawkGrips, but they all follow the same principle of using tools (typically stainless steel), breaking

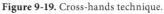

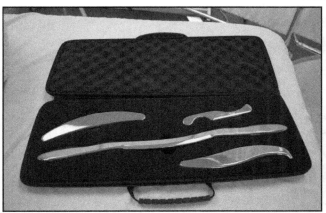

Figure 9-21. IASTM tools.

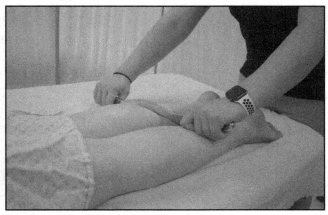

Figure 9-22. Therapist using tools on body part.

down scar tissue, releasing adhesions, and promoting improved mobility.[24] The tools are ergonomic and shaped to address different parts of the body to reduce strain on a therapist's hands when providing manual treatments, as well as to increase the pressure and focus of treatment to the patient's tissues. Figure 9-21 shows examples of IASTM tools. Typically, some type of emollient or lubricant is used with the tools to decrease bruising or discomfort during the treatment. Similar to myofascial techniques, IASTM involves the therapist moving across the muscle fibers (Figure 9-22). IASTM is thought to work by causing connective tissue remodeling by encouraging collagen repair and regeneration via fibroblast recruitment; this in turn may break down scar tissue and adhesions.[24] There is also the supposition that the action of using the tools increases the inflammatory response, inciting improved healing.[25] A physical therapist assistant can take continuing education classes to become certified in a specific type of IASTM techniques.

Joint Mobilizations

Joint mobilization is not always classified as a type of STM. Whereas STM or massage techniques are concerned with the movement of soft tissue (muscles, fascia, connective tissue), joint mobilization occurs when there is movement of joints and their supportive structures. Joint mobilization follows normal joint arthrokinematics, and there are specific guidelines and grades. Some suggest that a joint mobilization is most effective after massage or myofascial techniques when the soft tissue is relaxed.

A therapist performing joint mobilizations must recall the expected or normal end feels for a joint and be familiar with the arthrokinematics (such as the roll and glide of a joint) to perform joint mobilizations correctly. The therapist will need to remember the convex/concave rule for joint surfaces. Though in most states physical therapist assistants can perform most of the joint mobilizations, there are some states that prohibit all mobilizations by physical therapist assistants and others that prohibit

certain grades, such as grade V manipulations. One must be familiar with one's state's practice act to know what can or cannot be performed.

The specific types of joint mobilizations discussed here were promoted by G.D. Maitland, an Australian physiotherapist. There are other types of joint mobilization techniques one can learn, but when thinking or speaking of joint mobilization, the Maitland method is what typically comes to mind. Joint mobilizations are classified by the joint position, the direction of mobilization, the type of mobilization, the grade of mobilization, and the dosage (or frequency) of treatment. Grades are I to V and progress in intensity. Grade I is a small amplitude movement at the beginning of the joint's available ROM. Grade II is a large amplitude movement within the joint's available ROM. These 2 grades are classified as slow and smooth and of a short duration, perhaps 1 to 2 minutes, 1 to 2 times per session.[26] Grade III is a large amplitude movement that reaches the end ROM, and grade IV is a small amplitude movement at the very end of the ROM. These grades are sometimes described as being sharper or quicker in rhythm, performed for several minutes each time, several (>1 to 2 times) per session.[26] Grade V is a high-velocity thrust (sometimes called a *manipulation* vs a *mobilization*) of small amplitude at the end of the available ROM.[26] Grade V is not recommended to be performed more than 3 times over several sessions. Sometimes the mobilizations are also referred to or categorized as oscillations.[26] It is also worth noting that some joint mobilization grades are accompanied by a traction force. Figure 9-23 shows an example of joint mobilization to the finger. Table 9-6 discusses the specifics about joint mobilizations.

SAFETY CONCERNS

The important techniques for massage, such as hand washing, patient positioning, and therapist body mechanics, have now been discussed. One should also consider the contraindications for STM and ensure the patient is

Table 9-6	
Procedures for Applying Joint Mobilizations	
Equipment Needed	• Sheets, pillows • Treatment table/chair • Timer
Treatment/ Parameters	• Confirm patient does not have contraindications. • Determine optimal patient position—supine, prone, or seated. • Remove clothing and jewelry from area. • Ensure patient is relaxed and mobilizations will be passive (for patient). • Stabilize joint as needed. • Shorten lever arm and keep hands/fingers as close to joint being treated as possible. • Duration is variable. • Check with patient after treatment.
Safety Considerations	• Monitor patient's response (verbally and visually) during treatment session. • Avoid joint mobilizations if patient has bone disease, osteomyelitis, fracture, ligament rupture, or bone disease/cancer. • Therapist should adhere to proper body mechanics during treatment.
Advantages	• Inexpensive • Easy to apply once skill is mastered • Can reduce pain so patient can perform other activities
Disadvantages	• Difficult for some to assess joint mobility or end feel • May cause pain or muscle guarding in patient • Patient is unable to use extremity/body or perform activities during treatment

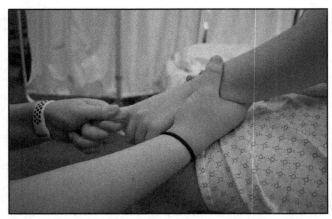

Figure 9-23. Joint mobilization being done on patient.

appropriate to receive the treatment. Clean thoroughly between each client; wipe down all surfaces and change the linens to avoid infection transmission. Confirm that the patient is not allergic to the lubricant being used or recommend the patient bring their own lubricant. Adjust the massage pressure and listen to the patient's feedback; provide patient education if the technique requires uncomfortable pressure. Finally, remember to encourage the patient to sit up slowly and sit on the edge of the bed or plinth for several minutes after treatment, especially if they have been prone or supine, because their blood pressure may drop initially on sitting, putting the patient as risk of falling. Remind the patient to hydrate well for the rest of the day, as this can also help.

DOCUMENTATION

When documenting STM or massage, first note what specific technique or method was used on the patient. Identify the location of treatment, patient position, and specific interventions performed. Also note the duration and frequency of treatment, as well as the patient response to treatment. See the following examples to get an idea of how to document these interventions.

Diagnosis: A female track runner presents with left patellar tendinitis as a result of repetitive motions and rates her pain during activity as 7/10 and at rest as 4/10. She has been taking 800 mg of ibuprofen every 8 hours and icing every 2 hours, but she still has pain.

O: Patient received transverse friction massage × 5 minutes to the left patellar tendon in the short seated position to place tendon on slight stretch. Patient reported discomfort during the treatment session but reported pain as 2/10 after session concluded. Ice applied to tendon after treatment × 15 minutes to decrease pain.

Diagnosis: Female, age 38 years, presents to therapy complaining that she "slept wrong" last night and now has significant pain in her upper neck and shoulders. She is unable to fully turn her head to the right without pain (ROM –18 degrees), rated at 6/10 with movement.

O: Patient received massage × 15 minutes to her upper neck and back, focusing on the upper trapezius and left sternocleidomastoid. Patient in prone with pillow under her lower extremities. Started with light effleurage and then progressed to petrissage using kneading and rolling to break up adhesions. Ended with another round of effleurage. Patient reported pain at 4/10 after session; ROM –10 degrees after session.

Conclusion

There are many types or examples of STM or massage, and each type has its own specific guidelines. Some techniques require certification and continuing education to perform them. In some states, physical therapist assistants are limited in what they can perform. Regardless of these variations, any type of STM aims to reduce swelling, improve pain, and promote improved mobility or ROM. There is some evidence that these techniques can also promote healing, improved immune response, and general relaxation or stress reduction.

Review Questions

1. Discuss the physiological effects of massage/STM.
2. What are 2 reflexive effects of massage?
3. Provide a massage technique that does not use lubricant.
4. Describe myofascial techniques and how they work on the tissues.
5. Provide 3 indications and 3 contraindications for STM.
6. When should effleurage be used during a massage intervention? Why?
7. List 5 considerations or guidelines when preparing to perform massage on a patient.
8. You have a patient complaining of pain that begins between the scapulae that radiates to their right shoulder. The pain is in a very specific location, and the patient reports that heat and medications have done little to help. What intervention might you recommend? Why? How would you document that intervention?

Case Study 1

Your patient is a 32-year-old woman who is having lower back pain and pain that radiates down her left leg after delivering a baby 10 weeks ago. She reports the pain is worse when carrying her baby or the baby carrier, and she feels some relief in supine. Your supervising physical therapist wants you to perform some STM to help alleviate pain and restore function.

1. What tissues are injured/affected?
2. What STM technique would you recommend for this patient? Why?
3. Describe the parameters and techniques you would use.
4. What are the contraindications for this treatment?
5. What other therapeutic modality would you recommend for this patient? Why?

Case Study 2

Your patient is a 42-year-old man who reports pain in his elbow, diagnosed as lateral epicondylitis. He has been icing the area as recommended by his physician, but the pain is still significant, a 7/10 with use of the elbow, and tender on palpation. He is an active weight lifter and would like to return to his routine as soon as possible.

1. What tissues are injured?
2. What STM technique(s) would you recommend for this patient? Why?
3. What other modality interventions would be appropriate for this patient? Why?
4. What are the parameters for the intervention?
5. What are the physiological effects of STM?

References

1. Jane SW, Chen SL, Wilkie DJ, et al. Effects of massage on pain, mood status, relaxation, and sleep in Taiwanese patients with metastatic bone pain: a randomized clinical trial. *Pain.* 2011;152(10):2432-2442.
2. Cherkin DC, Sherman KJ, Kahn J, et al. A comparison of the effects of 2 types of massage and usual care on chronic low back pain: a randomized controlled trial. *Ann Intern Med.* 2011;155(1):1-9.
3. Symons TB, Munk N, Shang Y, Cheng R, Yu G. Lower limb massage increases skeletal muscle blood flow in young women. *Med Sci Sports Exerc.* 2011;43(5):295.
4. Portillo-Soto A, Eberman LE, Demchak TJ, Peebles C. Comparison of blood flow changes with soft tissue mobilization and massage therapy. *J Altern Complement Med.* 2014;20(12):932-936.
5. Hilbert J, Sforzo G, Swensen T. The effects of massage on delayed onset muscle soreness. *Br J Sports Med.* 2003;37(1):72-75.

6. Smith LL, Keating MN, Holbert D, et al. The effects of athletic massage on delayed onset muscle soreness, creatine kinase, and neutrophil count: a preliminary report. *J Orthop Sports Phys Ther.* 1994;19(2):93-99.

7. Brod S, Rattazzi L, Piras G, D'Aquisto F. "As above, so below" examining the interplay between emotion and the immune system. *Immunology.* 2014;143(3):311-318.

8. Ang J, Lua J, Mathur A, et al. A randomized placebo-controlled trial of massage therapy on the immune system of preterm infants. *Pediatrics.* 2012;130(6):e1549-e1558.

9. Major B, Rattazzi L, Brod S, Pilipović I, Leposavić G, D'Acquisto F. Massage-like stroking boosts the immune system in mice. *Sci Rep.* 2015;5:10913.

10. Lovas JM, Craig AR, Segal YD, Raison RL, Weston KM, Markus MR. The effects of massage therapy on the human immune response in healthy adults. *J Bodyw Mov Ther.* 2002;6(3):143-150.

11. Hopper D, Conneely M, Chromiak F, Canini E, Berggren J, Briffa K. Evaluation of the effect of two massage techniques on hamstring muscle length in competitive female hockey players. *Phys Ther Sport.* 2005;6(3):137-145.

12. Patel K, Kobayashi M, Crawford S, et al. No. 63 Immediate massage stimulates muscle regeneration, angiogenesis, and decreases fibrosis after muscle injury. *Am J Phys Med Rehabil.* 2014;6(Suppl 8):S95.

13. Fernández-de-las-Peñas C, Alonso-Blanco C, Fernández-Carnero J, Miangolarra-Page J. The immediate effect of ischemic compression technique and transverse friction massage on tenderness of active and latent myofascial trigger points: a pilot study. *J Bodyw Mov Ther.* 2006;10(1):3-9.

14. Money S. Pathophysiology of trigger points in myofascial pain syndrome. *J Pain Palliat Care Pharmacolother.* 2017;31(2):158-159.

15. Andrzejewski W, Kassolik K, Dziegiel P, et al. Effects of synergistic massage and physical exercise on the expression of angiogenic markers in rat tendons. *Biomed Res Int.* 2014;2014:878095.

16. Wasserman J, Steele-Thornborrow J, Yuen J, Halkiotis M, Riggens E, Chronic caesarian section scar pain treated with fascial scar release techniques: a case series. *J Bodyw Mov Ther.* 2016;20(4):906-913.

17. Haun JN, Graham-Pole J, Shortley B. Children with cancer and blood diseases experience positive physical and psychological effects from massage therapy. *Int J Ther Massage Bodywork.* 2009;2(2):7-14.

18. Richards KC, Gibson R, Overton-McCoy AL. Effects of massage in acute and critical care. *AACN Clin Issues.* 2000;11(1):77-96.

19. Hsu WC, Guo SE, Chang CH. Back massage intervention for improving health and sleep quality among intensive care unit patients. *Nurs Crit Care.* 2019;24(5):313-319.

20. Westman KF, Blaisdell C. CE: many benefits, little risk: the use of massage in nursing practice. *Am J Nurs.* 2016;116(1):34-39.

21. Hoffa A. *Technik der Massage.* Verlag Vox Ferdinand Enke; 1893.

22. Chamberlain GJ. Cyriax's friction massage: a review. *J Orthop Sports Phys Ther.* 1982;4(1):16-22.

23. Kukadia H, Malshikare A, Palekar T. Effect of passive stretching v/s myofascial release in improving piriformis flexibility in females—a comparative study. *Indian J Physiother Occup Ther.* 2019;13(4):57-61.

24. Cheatham SW, Lee M, Cain M, Baker R. The efficacy of instrument assisted soft tissue mobilization: a systematic review. *J Can Chiropr Assoc.* 2016;60(3):200-211.

25. Kim J, Sung DJ, Lee J. Therapeutic effectiveness of instrument-assisted soft tissue mobilization for soft tissue injury: mechanisms and practical application. *J Exerc Rehabil.* 2017;13(1):12-22.

26. Hengeveld E, Banks K, eds. *Maitland's Peripheral Manipulation: Management of Neuromusculoskeletal Disorders.* Vol. 2. 5th ed. Churchill Livingstone–Elsevier; 2013.

Unit V

Electrical Agents

Chapter 10

Electrotherapy

KEY TERMS Absolute refractory period | Accommodation | Action potential | Alternating current | Ampere | Amplitude | Anode | Biphasic current | Cathode | Conductors | Current | Depolarization | Direct current | Frequency | Impedance | Insulators | Monophasic current | Ohm | Overload principle | Phase duration | Propagation | Pulsatile current | Pulse duration | Repolarization | Resistance | Resting membrane potential | Specificity | Sweep | Voltage | Watt | Waveforms

KEY ABBREVIATIONS HVPC | IFC | NMES | PENS | Pre-Mod | TENS

CHAPTER OBJECTIVES

1. Describe electrotherapy and its different techniques.
2. Be able to define the different types of currents and waveforms.
3. Discuss the physiological effects of electrotherapy, including how electrical current moves through the body's tissues.
4. Discuss the guidelines and considerations for the application of electrotherapy as physical therapy interventions.
5. Explain the indications and contraindications for electrotherapy interventions.
6. Demonstrate adherence to safety when applying electrical modalities.
7. Apply knowledge of electrotherapy set-up and parameters to case scenarios.
8. Document electrotherapy interventions correctly in a patient's chart.

INTRODUCTION

Richard Holmes writes in his book *Age of Wonder: The Romantic Generation and the Discovery of the Beauty and Terror of Science* that the use of electricity to stimulate muscles was discovered, in part, when Luigi Galvani hooked (disembodied) frog legs up to an electrical current; his nephew, Giovanni Aldini, took it a step further and tried the same on corpses to see if they would come back to life.[1] Sound familiar? Interestingly, these events coincided with Mary Shelley's writing of *Frankenstein; or, The Modern Prometheus*, and is thought to have inspired the reanimation of Frankenstein's creature in the book.

While clinicians now know that electricity cannot, generally, bring the dead to life (although the use of an automatic external defibrillator comes pretty close), it can provide other benefits. To understand how electricity provides these benefits, one must first understand certain terminology, the currents and waveforms, and the basic parameters of electrotherapy.

CURRENT AND WAVEFORM TYPES

Electricity has quite a few terms in reference to how it is measured and how it moves. The rate at which electrical current flows is called an *ampere* (A, amp), and an electrical current flow is described in units of milliamperes, denoted as mA, or in microamperes, denoted as µA. Amps are considered to represent the amount of electricity flowing. Ohm is the measure of resistance; the higher the resistance, the lower the flow (amperes) and vice versa. Voltage (volt) is what makes electric charges move, and the electrons move from an area of higher electrons to lower electrons.

Memolo J.
Therapeutic Agents for the Physical Therapist Assistant
(pp 115-138). © 2022 SLACK Incorporated.

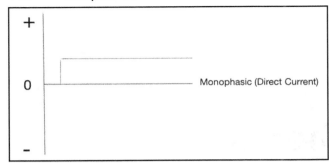

Figure 10-1. Monophasic drawing.

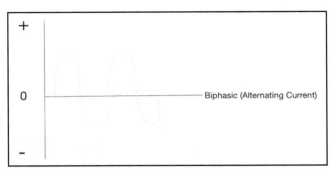

Figure 10-2. Biphasic drawing.

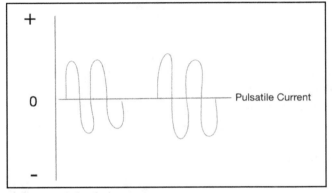

Figure 10-3. Pulsatile drawing.

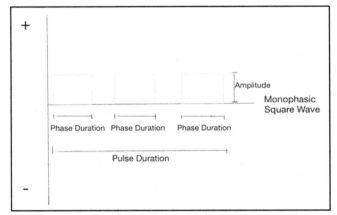

Figure 10-4. Waveform example.

To help understand this better, one might think of water flowing through a pipe; volts correlate to a water pump (the thing that makes the water move); amps are like the amount of water flowing, such as gallons or liters; and ohms correlate to the diameter and smoothness of the pipe the water is flowing through (the smaller the diameter, the higher the resistance). The amount of electrical power generated is measured as a watt, so this is similar to the power flowing water produces as a product of the number of gallons or liters flowing (amps) and the pressure created by the pipe (volts).

It is also important to understand that electricity flows best with good conductors. *Conductance* is the term used to describe the ease with which a current flow along a medium; it is measured in siemens. Good conductors include metals or electrolyte solutions (eg, electricity flows well through water). Materials that do now allow electricity to flow easily are called *insulators*, and examples include wood, glass, air, and in the human body, fat tissue.

Electrotherapy devices generally create 3 different currents that can cause physiological changes in the tissue. These currents are monophasic or direct current (DC), biphasic or alternating current (AC), and pulsatile current (PC). Monophasic currents, sometimes also called *galvanic currents*, have a unidirectional flow of electrons toward the positive pole or negative pole (Figure 10-1). Biphasic currents have electron flow that reverses polarity, or in other words, changes directions from positive to negative

(Figure 10-2). PCs have several pulses grouped together that can be unidirectional or bidirectional and the groups are interrupted (Figure 10-3).

It may be helpful to understand the various waveforms, which are basically the picture representation of the shape, direction, amplitude, duration, and pulse frequency of the electrical current being generated by the electrotherapeutic device. It is a way to visualize the electrical current. Waveforms can be sinusoidal, rectangular, square, or spiked. Figure 10-4 shows a monophasic square phase, and Figure 10-5 shows a biphasic spiked wave. Waveforms will be addressed in the next section as a part of electrotherapy parameters.

PARAMETER MODULATION

Electrical stimulation modalities require the adjustment of a few basic parameters to achieve the desired goal. The specifics of these settings will be discussed later, but this section will talk about what the parameters are.

As mentioned earlier, the waveform is the representation of the direction, amplitude, duration, and pulse frequency of the current being generated. Some may consider the waveform to be the type or name of electrical stimulation provided. One may also see a term such as *current modulation*, with examples being continuous or burst. A

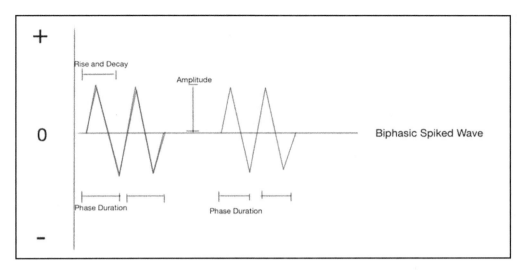

Figure 10-5. Waveform example.

continuous current is one that has the same current flow for a period of time, whereas a burst setting has a short duration of current that turns on and off (in bursts).

Pulse frequency, measured as pulses per second (pps), is another parameter to set on an electrical stimulation unit. In some cases, one might see this also measured in hertz (Hz) or see it called *pulse rate*. This represents the type of muscle response to expect from the treatment. A low frequency will yield individual twitches or contractions in a muscle; the closer together the twitches (and thus the higher the frequency), the more the twitches begin to resemble one tetanic contraction. As frequency increases, so does the likelihood of muscle fatigue.

Pulse or phase duration is measured in microseconds (μs) and represents the length of time an electrical current is flowing during one cycle. In some units, the pulse duration is set at a fixed rate; shorter pulse durations tend to be more comfortable for patients if the number is adjustable. Longer pulse durations may be required to achieve an action potential.

Amplitude, which also means the electrical stimulation intensity, will generally indicate the strength of the muscle contraction or stimulation desired. Amplitude can be measured in amperes (A), microamperes (μA), or milliamperes (mA). The amplitude must be increased enough to yield either a sensory stimulation or a muscle contraction, but the exact numbers for these differ based on the goal and the patient.

On and off times are used in certain electrical stimulation protocols and are needed to reduce the amount of fatigue a muscle experiences as a result of the intervention. The on time is the amount of time the electrical stimulation is on and stimulating the muscle, and the off time, which is either equal to or sometimes longer than the on time, is the time the electrical stimulation is not on. This should not be confused with the ramp time, which is a time set to allow the electrical stimulation to build up to its maximal amplitude. It would not be ideal for the electrical current to suddenly turn on at maximum amplitude and contract or stimulate a muscle; this would be uncomfortable. The ramp time (up and down) allows the current to gradually reach peak amplitude and then gradually decrease again.

Finally, one needs to adjust treatment time (per treatment) and treatment frequency (per day or week). As one might expect, these numbers vary according to the type of intervention, the goals of that intervention, and the patient response. When using electrical stimulation to strengthen a muscle, for example, one may measure the duration in terms of how many muscle contractions are desired, and one must consider that the targeted muscle will fatigue. Other treatments for pain reduction may be used for up to 24 hours/day, as needed.

There are a few other parameters one might see in specific electrical stimulation settings, such as beat frequency (specific to interferential current [IFC]) or polarity (specific to DC in the treatment of wounds, edema, or in the case of iontophoresis). It is also important to consider electrode placement, but this will be discussed specifically with each type of intervention.

PHYSIOLOGICAL EFFECTS OF ELECTROTHERAPY

Before learning about the different types of electrical stimulation, one must understand the potential physiological effects of electrical current on biological tissues. Generally, one can divide the physiological effects into nerve, tissue, and muscle responses.

Nerve Responses to Electrical Modalities

To understand how electrical currents affect nerves, one must first understand how a nerve is stimulated. A nerve at rest has a more negative charge inside (with potassium ions) than outside (with sodium ions); this is called the nerve's

Figure 10-6. Action potential drawing.

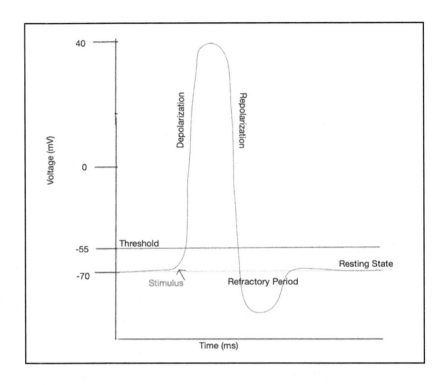

resting membrane potential and is the cell's normal homeostatic state. A strong enough stimulus (such as an electrical current) opens the sodium channels in the cell membrane and causes the inside of the cell to become more positively charged. This depolarizes the cell membrane. Once the cell membrane reaches a certain threshold, the potassium channels open and the cell is repolarized. This depolarization and repolarization is called an *action potential*, which is the basic way a nerve communicates.

What this all amounts to is that electrical stimulation must generate a stimulus that meets a certain threshold; doing so will change the cell membrane's permeability and thus cause an action potential, which sends an impulse along the nerve. Unless the electrical stimulation is sufficient in duration and intensity, an action potential will not be fired and there will be no sensory stimulus or muscle contraction (depending on what one wants). Figure 10-6 shows a visual representation of an action potential.

Once a nerve is depolarized, no other action potentials can be generated, no matter how strong the stimulus might be. Think of it as the nerve being fatigued and needing to rest. This is called the *absolute refractory period*. When an action potential is generated, it can trigger action potentials down the line in adjacent areas; this is called *propagation* along the neuron. The speed of nerve conduction depends on the size or diameter of the nerve and the nerve's myelination. Sometimes, a patient will accommodate to the stimulation because the nerve eventually becomes less sensitive to the current. Once the nerve returns to its resting membrane potential, then another action potential can be generated.

Something else to think about is the strength-duration curve. What this represents is the amount of electrical current required to produce an action potential in specific types of nerves. Chapter 1 discussed Aβ sensory fibers and Aδ and C fibers for pain sensations. The strength-duration curve shows the amplitude and pulse duration required to stimulate each of these nerve fibers, as well as motor nerve fibers. Essentially, low-amplitude and short-pulse durations are sufficient to stimulate sensory Aβ nerves; higher amplitudes and longer durations are required to yield a muscle contraction; even higher amplitudes and longer pulses are needed to depolarize C fibers (although C fibers can be stimulated at low durations with a high enough amplitude); and highest amplitudes and longest pulses are required to stimulate denervated muscle nerves. The higher the amplitudes and the longer the pulse durations, the more uncomfortable the stimulation typically will be. Figure 10-7 shows a picture of the strength-duration curve.

This ties back to the Gate Control theory and the Opiate theory for pain control. Certain settings of electrotherapeutic modalities will stimulate those Aβ fibers (the superficial sensory fibers) and can close the gate for pain sensations in the brain. If the stimulation is stronger and more noxious, the brain may make natural endogenous opiates as a response, causing a more long-term pain reduction.

Tissue Responses to Electrical Modalities

While it is not completely known by what mechanism(s) electrical stimulation promotes wound healing, and the set parameters for wound healing are not clear, clinical studies

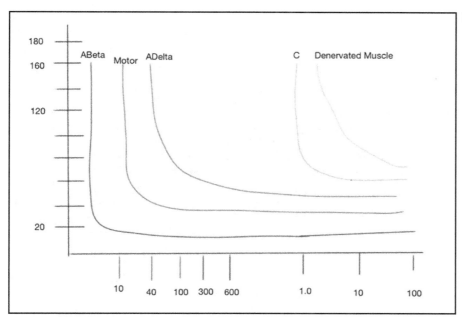

Figure 10-7. Strength-duration curve.

do support that it is an effective treatment.[2-4] Studies indicate that wound healing occurs as a result of attracting cells specific to healing, such as neutrophils, macrophages, lymphocytes, and fibroblasts, to the wound area, possibly via the electrical charge.[5] Other research indicates that wound healing is promoted by fibroblast replication and DNA synthesis brought on by the electrical stimulation.[5] Electrical stimulation may also suppress the expression of certain genes responsible for inflammation; too much inflammation may prevent the wound from progressing to the proliferative phase, and so a reduction of inflammation may promote improved wound healing.[6]

The use of electrical stimulation to treat edema is questionable; depending on the study one reads, the outcomes vary. Some argue that there is no statistical significance between edema treated with electrical stimulation and edema treated otherwise[7,8]; a recent systematic review of studies indicates that edema can be successfully treated with electrical stimulation.[9] The most obvious way electrical stimulation might help reduce edema is by replicating our normal muscle pump. If you think about how veins work, the compression of the muscles around the veins help push or pump fluid back up toward the heart. The veins have valves to prevent any backflow. If a patient is unable to activate their lower extremity muscles, that pump is hindered and fluid may collect. Electrical stimulation that causes the muscles to contract can simulate what normally occurs and pump fluid back up toward the heart.

Less agreed-on is the idea that the use of electrical charge, specifically a negative charge using a high-voltage pulsed current (HVPC), may repel proteins and accelerate their uptake by lymphatic capillaries, thus reducing the interstitial fluid.[10] In addition, some research suggests this negative charge promotes lymphatic flow and drainage.[10]

However, more recent research varies on its verdict regarding this methodology. A 2010 systematic review indicated that it might reduce edema in this way,[11] but other studies are less certain.

Another potential use for electrical stimulation is to promote bone growth, and its use to stimulate bone healing in otherwise nonhealing fractures is fairly well documented.[12] Like wound healing and edema reduction, electrical stimulation's effects on bone repair are not well understood, although studies have shown the formation of a bone callus with electrical stimulation. Like the research with wound healing, studies of electrical stimulation's effects on bone show that it stimulates the "synthesis of growth factors, collagen synthesis, proteoglycans, and cytokines."[13]

Muscle Responses to Electrical Modalities

As mentioned previously, muscle nerves can be depolarized and yield an action potential, which can result in a muscle contraction. This is how normal, innervated muscle contractions work. In an innervated muscle, an action potential must be met to achieve a muscle contraction. Once that depolarizing threshold is met, the muscle contraction occurs regardless of the strength of the stimulus. This is called the *all-or-none response*. Basically, the stimulus either meets the threshold and causes the depolarization or it does not; there is no in between.

Denervated muscles, or those that have lost their peripheral nerve supply, are more difficult to stimulate than innervated muscles and require different parameters. Denervated muscles lack function, experience atrophy, and are eventually replaced by fibrous connective tissue[14] if the nerves do not regenerate. Stimulation of denervated muscles aims to reduce or slow the speed of this atrophy, and this is especially important if the nerve has the potential to regenerate. Some studies indicate that stimulating denervated muscles may improve or promote the regeneration of nerve axons,[15] and that electrical stimulation is beneficial even to permanently denervated muscles such as in the case of spinal cord injuries.[16] As mentioned previously, the amplitude and pulse duration to stimulate a denervated muscle are much higher and longer than those required to provide sensory or innervated muscle motor stimulation. The purpose is to depolarize not the nerve cell membrane, but rather the muscle membrane itself.

ELECTRICAL STIMULATION FOR DRUG DELIVERY

Iontophoresis is the use of DC to deliver an ionically charged drug transdermally. The treatment uses the concept of polarity (in that like charges repel) to push or drive a drug through the skin and into the tissue, sometimes called *electromigration*.[17] Another mechanism for drug delivery is that of electro-osmosis, or the movement of liquids across the tissue due to the electrical charge.[17] Still others believe that electrical current makes the outermost layer of the skin, the stratum corneum, more permeable.

ELECTRICAL STIMULATION BIOFEEDBACK

All physiological effects discussed thus far relate to how electricity enters the body and then causes certain outcomes. In the case of electromyographic (EMG) biofeedback, electrical current does not enter the tissue. Rather, electrodes are placed on the muscle belly and provide information on how that muscle is contracting; it reads the electrical current being generated by that muscle. Specifically, EMG biofeedback picks up on the action potentials occurring in the area. The information received, which can be interpreted through a machine via audio, visual, or a combination of feedback methods, allows the patient to see (or hear) how the muscle is performing and, in this way, the patient can be motivated to either contract or relax a muscle, depending on the desired outcome. If a patient has too much muscle guarding, for example, the machine will beep or light up; a patient can consciously attempt to relax that muscle to make the noise and lights go away. In this way, a side effect (or secondary effect) may be a reduction of pain.

INDICATIONS AND CONTRAINDICATIONS OF ELECTROTHERAPY

So far, this chapter has described when and how one might use electrical stimulation on a patient, but this section will look at the specific indications and contraindications for this modality.

Muscle contraction is the most obvious clinical application for electrical stimulation. There are a variety of reasons to initiate a muscle contraction; the most common are to strengthen a muscle, to stimulate a denervated muscle for muscle re-education or to decrease atrophy, or to increase range of motion. Electrical stimulation can fatigue a muscle, so it can be helpful in treating muscle spasms or muscle guarding or to reduce increased muscle tone. Making a muscle contract and move could also help reduce edema (and increase circulation) by simulating the normal muscle pump similar to when a patient performs active movement.

Other indications for electrical stimulation include reduction of pain. Either via the Gate Control theory or the Opiate theory, electrical stimulation can reduce pain, which can allow a patient to perform more or better-quality exercises and therapeutic activities as well as perform activities of daily living.

Additionally, electrical stimulation is used to heal wounds and fractures. The use of electricity in the form of iontophoresis can deliver a drug through the skin to help decrease pain or inflammation. Finally, EMG biofeedback reads the electrical activity in a muscle and can then be used to help relax muscle guarding or contract a weak muscle to help with muscle re-education.

While electrical stimulation can lead to many beneficial outcomes, one must ensure the patient does not have any contraindications. These include if the patient has a pacemaker because the electrical current could disrupt the function of the device. One should not apply electrical stimulation over the carotid artery; fluid with electrolytes is a great conductor of electricity, and this placement could negatively affect blood pressure and heart rate. Pregnant patients are generally contraindicated for all forms of electrical stimulation, although some might suggest not applying electrical stimulation over the abdomen or low back area. In some cases, transcutaneous electrical nerve stimulation (TENS) is used during labor to decrease back pain, and this has been determined to be safe for this short period. As always, if the patient has a known or suspected deep vein thrombosis or thrombophlebitis, no electrical stimulation should be used lest it dislodge the clot and cause an embolus.

Other precautions to applying electrical stimulation to a patient include cardiac disease, patients with cancer, patients with impaired cognition, and patients with impaired or absent sensation. Unless one is administering electrical stimulation to specifically heal a wound, avoid placing electrodes over open areas of skin because the electrical current can unevenly disperse in the tissue and cause burns. Table 10-1 lists all of the indications, contraindications, and physiological effects of electrical stimulation.

Table 10-1

Indications, Contraindications, and Physiological Effects of Electrical Stimulation

Indications	Contraindications	Physiological Effects
Wound care	Pacemaker	Nerve stimulation via nerve depolarization and action potential
Edema reduction	Over the carotid artery	All-or-none response of muscle
Muscle strengthening	Pregnancy (especially over the lower back or abdomen)	Muscle membrane depolarization (for denervated nerves)
Muscle re-education	Deep vein thrombosis	Gate Control theory
Prevent muscle atrophy	Cardiac disease (precaution)	Opiate theory
Reduce muscle guarding	Cancer (precaution)	Attracts cells specific to healing
Reduce muscle spasm	Impaired cognition/sensation (precaution)	Fibroblast replication and DNA synthesis
Increase range of motion	Over open areas unless specifically performing wound care (precaution)	Use of polarity to repel proteins and promote lymphatic flow
Heal fractures/tendons/ligaments	Eyes	Stimulates bone growth factors, collagen synthesis, proteoglycans, and cytokines
Stimulate nerve regeneration	Gonads	Deliver drugs transdermally via electromigration, electro-osmosis, and increasing skin permeability
Reduce pain		Use of EMG biofeedback to "read" muscle activity

APPLICATION METHODS

This section will discuss the variety of ways to apply electrical current to a patient for therapeutic purposes. There are a variety of units and devices to administer electrical stimulation; some units also have a combination of modalities such as ultrasound or laser. Figures 10-8 through 10-10 offer some examples of these units. Bear in mind that while parameters are included here, they can vary and one may see other clinicians using slightly different parameters in their treatment.

Sensory-Level Electrical Stimulation

While the use of electricity to stimulate muscle contractions seems the most obvious use of electrical current, the other most common use of electrical stimulation is to decrease pain. These are commonly used techniques in the clinic, but at-home units are also available at the local drug store. Devices used in the clinic are different from the over-the-counter versions and require the clinician to understand the physiological effects, the contraindications, as well as the specifics on how to adjust the parameters to get the desired outcome.

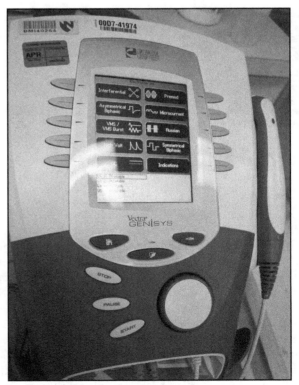

Figure 10-8. Chattanooga unit.

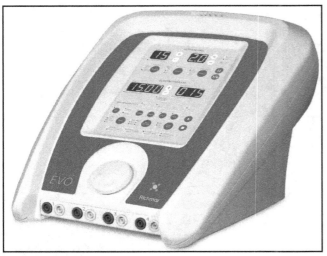

Figure 10-9. Unit with combination—Mettler.

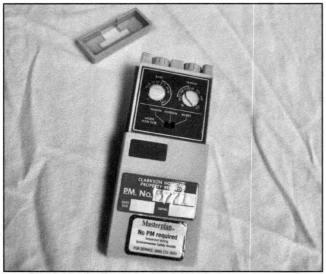

Figure 10-11. TENS unit.

Transcutaneous Electrical Nerve Stimulation

A TENS unit is a frequently used device to help reduce pain in the clinic. Figure 10-11 shows an example of a TENS unit. Benefits include making pain manageable for the patient leading up to or following a therapy treatment session, but it is important to note that a TENS unit can also be worn during the treatment session. However TENS is used, it can allow patients to be more active during their therapy session and have pain relief after the session. TENS units can also be sent home with the patient (after proper education, of course), so that the patient can wear the device during the day when needed. TENS relieves pain, but the way it accomplishes this varies depending on the settings.

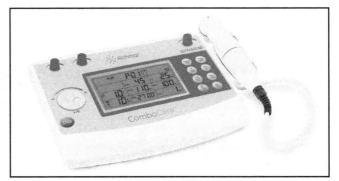

Figure 10-10. Unit with combo—Combo care.

Most units have 3 setting options: conventional, acupuncture, or burst.

Conventional, or high-frequency, TENS works by stimulating the superficial sensory nerves (the Aβ fibers) and thus close the gate for pain (the Gate Control theory). Pain is modulated while the patient wears the unit, but the effects are short-lived or limited only to when the patient is wearing the unit. While most treatment sessions last about 30 minutes, a patient can wear the unit and use conventional TENS all day if needed. However, the patient will accommodate to the treatment, and the intensity may have to be increased to receive the same level of pain relief. This means a therapist may advise the patient to instead use the TENS when needed, such as when walking or performing a painful daily activity, like gardening. Often, the patient will apply the electrodes at the beginning of the day and then turn on the unit as needed.

Acupuncture TENS, also sometimes called *low-frequency TENS*, has an intensity high enough to elicit a muscle contraction, and the sensation is described by some as strong but not painful. Acupuncture TENS is thought to work by depolarizing the Aδ and C fibers by activating the descending pain mechanisms that originate in the brainstem.[18] Unlike conventional TENS, acupuncture TENS is not appropriate to wear for longer periods of time, perhaps 20 to 30 minutes, but the pain-relieving effects may last up to an hour or 2 after the unit is turned off.

Finally, burst TENS is considered a noxious stimulus, and thus reduces pain via the Gate Control and the Opiate theories. The settings have both a high intensity and a high frequency, and as a result burst TENS affects both the Aβ and Aδ fibers. The patient may report a sensory feeling similar to that of getting a tattoo (a prickly sensation).[19] This noxious stimulus may stimulate the release of natural endorphins and, as a result, the treatment duration should not exceed 15 minutes because the patient likely will not tolerate much longer than that. However, because burst TENS works via the Gate Control and Opiate theories, the pain relief felt from treatment may last several hours. Table 10-2 discusses the set-up for TENS treatments, and Table 10-3 lists the parameters for each TENS setting.[19,20]

Table 10-2	
Procedures for Applying Transcutaneous Electrical Nerve Stimulation	
Equipment Needed	• TENS unit • Electrodes • Wires • Alcohol wipes • Sheets, pillows • Treatment table/chair • Timer
Treatment/ Parameters	• Confirm patient does not have contraindications. • Determine optimal patient position—supine, prone, or seated. • Remove clothing and jewelry from area. • Prepare skin area prior to electrode placement—clean with alcohol wipe, trim excessive hair, ensure skin is intact, etc. • Apply electrodes and connect to unit via wires. • Establish correct parameters for TENS treatment. • Turn on unit and monitor patient's response. Let unit run for a few cycles before leaving the patient (if you are doing so). • Make sure patient has a call bell if you are leaving patient alone. • Check patient's skin and ask for feedback after treatment.
Safety Considerations	• Monitor patient's response (verbally and visually) during treatment session. • Make sure skin prep is done before applying electrodes.
Advantages	• Portable units can be relatively inexpensive • Patient can perform therapy interventions while connected to unit • Can reduce pain so patient can perform other activities
Disadvantages	• Larger units are more expensive • Can be difficult for patients to self-administer safely or correctly • Patient can accommodate to intensity over time • Some pain relief may be temporary, requiring more frequent use

Table 10-3					
Transcutaneous Electrical Nerve Stimulation Parameters					
TENS Type	pps (Pulse Frequency)[19,20]	Pulse Duration (μs)[19,20]	Amplitude (Intensity) in mA	Duration	How It Works
Conventional	30 to 150	50 to 100	To tingling	≤ 24 hours as needed	Gate Control theory
Acupuncture	2 to 5	100 to 300	Tingling, muscle twitch	20 to 45 min	Descending Pain theory
Burst	Preset; 2 to 10 bursts; 60 to 100	150 to 500	To noxious stimulus or motor response	≤ 15 min as tolerated	Gate Control and Opiate theories

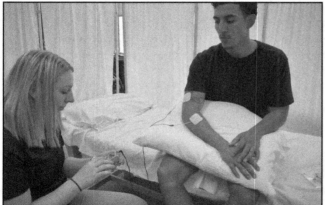

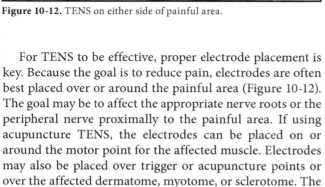

Figure 10-12. TENS on either side of painful area.

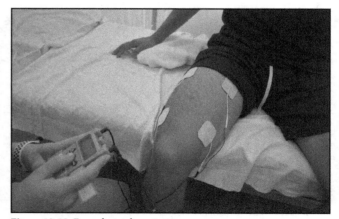

Figure 10-13. Four electrodes set-up.

For TENS to be effective, proper electrode placement is key. Because the goal is to reduce pain, electrodes are often best placed over or around the painful area (Figure 10-12). The goal may be to affect the appropriate nerve roots or the peripheral nerve proximally to the painful area. If using acupuncture TENS, the electrodes can be placed on or around the motor point for the affected muscle. Electrodes may also be placed over trigger or acupuncture points or over the affected dermatome, myotome, or sclerotome. The clinician can choose to use 2 or 4 electrodes as needed. Figure 10-13 shows a quadripolar pad placement for TENS.

Interferential and Premodulated Current

IFC gets its name from the fact that this setting uses 2 currents that interfere with each other. Recall from the acupuncture TENS discussion that low-frequency electrical stimulation can yield pain during treatment; this is because the skin offers more impedance to low-frequency current.[21] IFC bypasses this by having one current at a lower frequency and one at a higher frequency, and these 2 currents interfere with each other. Thus, IFC can result in more long-term pain reduction to deeper tissues while avoiding the discomfort felt during the treatment.[21-23] This is one of the benefits of using IFC vs TENS for pain relief. Another benefit is that IFC allows the clinician to address pain in a large area.

Similar to conventional TENS, IFC is thought to offer pain relief via the Gate Control theory, although the use of the low-frequency setting may also work via the Opiate theory.[21] Some other studies support the use of IFC for muscle stimulation, edema reduction[8] (likely via the aforementioned muscle stimulation), or for the treatment of stress incontinence when combined with Kegel exercises,[24] although some of these studies vary in their opinions about how well IFC addresses these concerns.

Usually, patients receive IFC from machines or units that have a specific IFC setting. Parameters include intensity and treatment time, but they also include a beat frequency and sweep settings that makes IFC unique. Intensity is usually increased until the patient reports a pleasant tingling sensation, and duration usually falls between 20 and 30 minutes. The beat frequency is the difference between the 2 current frequencies used in the treatment. For example, if one current is 4000 Hz (or pps) and the other is 3800 Hz, the beat frequency would be 200 Hz. One might decide what beat frequency to select based on the goal of the treatment. If the aim is pain relief similar to conventional TENS, the beat frequency may fall between 50 and 130 Hz. If acupuncture TENS–type pain relief is the goal, 2 to 5 pps would be the beat frequency selection. If the aim is to yield a muscle contraction, the beat frequency may be closer to 20 to 50 Hz. Some machines allow the clinician to specifically adjust the frequencies or select the beat frequency; others have this preset or limit the options. The sweep setting is a way to prevent nerves from accommodating to the stimulation. The sweep means the frequency slightly changes, or sweeps within a range, to avoid accommodation. The clinician can choose whether the settings will be fixed or in a sweep setting. Some units allow for 2 to 3 preset options: a narrow sweep between 2 smaller numbers, such as between 5 and 10 Hz (pps); a wide sweep between a larger number, such as between 1 and 250 Hz (pps); and a medium sweep, such as between 80 and 150 Hz (pps). The wider the range of the sweep, the more the patient might feel and/or the less they may accommodate to the treatment. Some machines also allow the clinician to adjust the time the sweep occurs, so one may set the unit to sweep between the 2 frequencies within 7 or 20 seconds. Table 10-4 lists the details of applying IFC to a patient, and Table 10-5 lists the parameters for IFC. Figure 10-14 shows a typical IFC parameter set-up on a unit, and Figure 10-15 shows a different IFC unit.

A final important point is the placement of the electrodes. Because true IFC uses 2 frequencies, this necessitates the use of 4 electrodes (quadripolar; 2 for each current). Additionally, because the goal is for the 2 currents to interfere with each other within the tissue, the electrodes must be placed surrounding the body part in question and crisscrossed. This will result in the maximum pain relief in

Table 10-4

Procedures for Applying Interferential Current

Equipment Needed	• Electrical stimulation unit with IFC setting • Electrodes • Wires • Alcohol wipes • Sheets, pillows • Treatment table/chair • Timer
Treatment/ Parameters	• Confirm patient does not have contraindications. • Determine optimal patient position—supine, prone, or seated. • Remove clothing and jewelry from area. • Prepare skin area before electrode placement—clean with alcohol wipe, trim excessive hair, ensure skin is intact, etc. • Apply electrodes and connect to unit via wires. • Establish the correct parameters for IFC treatment. • Turn on unit and monitor patient's response. Let unit run for a few cycles before leaving the patient (if you are doing so). • Make sure patient has a call bell if you are leaving patient alone. • Check patient's skin and ask for feedback after treatment.
Safety Considerations	• Monitor patient's response (verbally and visually) during treatment session. • Make sure skin prep is done before applying electrodes.
Advantages	• Patient may be able to perform therapy interventions while connected to unit • Can reduce pain so patient can perform other activities after treatment
Disadvantages	• Larger units are more expensive • Patient can accommodate to intensity over time unless sweep setting used • Some pain relief may be temporary, requiring more frequent use

Table 10-5

Interferential Current Parameters

	pps (Pulse Frequency)	Amplitude (Intensity) in mA	Duration	Modulation	How It Works
IFC	Beat frequency: 2 to 10, 1 to 250, 80 to 150 (low, medium, and high)	To a comfortable tingling sensation	20 to 30 min	Sweep or fixed	Gate Control theory, Opiate theory

the area where the 2 currents intersect. Electrodes should not be too close to each other to avoid the risk of burns, and larger electrodes may be more comfortable for the patient. See Figure 10-16 for an IFC electrode configuration.

Premodulated IFC, or premodulated current, is similar to true IFC in most ways; the goal is to generally address pain or possibly produce muscle contractions. The difference is that the current frequencies are mixed inside the unit and then delivered through one channel (one pair of electrodes or a bipolar electrode configuration) rather than them interfering in the tissue via 4 electrodes.

Motor-Level Electrical Stimulation

This section focuses on the use of electrical stimulation to produce muscle contractions. The indications section listed the various reasons one might want to do this,

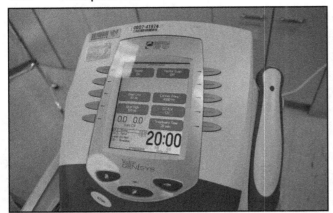

Figure 10-14. IFC parameter set-up on unit.

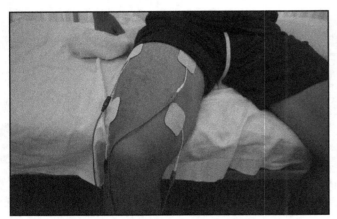

Figure 10-16. IFC crisscrossed electrodes.

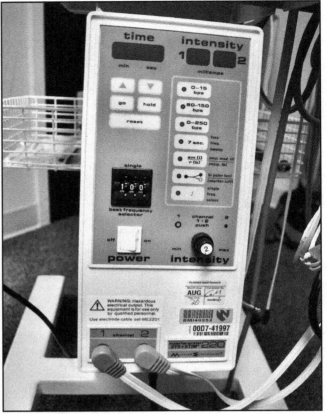

Figure 10-15. IFC unit.

namely, to increase muscle strength, prevent muscle atrophy, re-educate muscles, reduce edema, decrease muscle guarding or spasms, and increase range of motion. In this section, the focus will be on the broad category of neuromuscular electrical stimulation (NMES) and its subsets.

Neuromuscular Electrical Stimulation

NMES depolarizes a muscle nerve (in innervated muscles) and the muscle itself (in denervated muscles), causing an action potential and a resulting contraction. However, there are a few differences between muscle contractions elicited by electrical stimulation and those initiated physiologically. As mentioned previously in the parameters section, NMES settings require an on/off time because electrically stimulated muscles fatigue quickly. This is in part because fast-twitch muscle fibers (type II) are stimulated first when electrical stimulation is used; normal physiological muscle contractions stimulate the slow-twitch fibers (type I) first, with the fast-twitch fibers recruited later. These type II fibers fatigue more quickly than the type I fibers. As a result, the off time should be longer than the on time to prolong the treatment time before fatigue sets in.

Another difference is that physiological contractions have a gradual or smooth onset, whereas those caused by electrical stimulation are more rapid and irregular. This is due to the motor units being stimulated all at once when the action potential threshold is met. The reason for the ramp time parameter is that it allows for a more gradual, comfortable contraction.

NMES is thought to strengthen muscles via 2 principles: the Overload principle and the Specificity theory. The Overload principle is one that applies to normal exercise as well as electrical stimulation; the greater the load placed on the muscle and the higher force of contractions, the stronger the muscle will be.[25] In normal exercise, this would happen with the increase of weight. In NMES, the muscle is simulated by increasing the intensity or amplitude of the current, thus increasing the force of the contraction. The Specificity theory relates to the aforementioned recruitment of type II, fast-twitch muscle fibers before type I fibers when using electrical stimulation. It suggests that, for this reason, electrical stimulation will have more of an effect on those fiber types.[26]

One aspect of an NMES treatment that varies according to the patient diagnosis and treatment protocol is to advise the patient to perform isometric muscle contractions of the muscle being stimulated simultaneously with the electrical stimulus.[27] In this way, patients are not passive

Table 10-6	
Procedures for Applying Neuromuscular Electrical Stimulation	
Equipment Needed	• Electrical stimulation unit • Electrodes • Wires • Alcohol wipes • Sheets, pillows • Treatment table/chair • Timer
Treatment/ Parameters	• Confirm patient does not have contraindications. • Determine optimal patient position—supine, prone, or seated. • Remove clothing and jewelry from area. • Prepare skin area before electrode placement—clean with alcohol wipe, trim excessive hair, ensure skin is intact, etc. • Apply electrodes and connect to unit via wires. If goal is to simulate a muscle pump for edema reduction, 2 electrodes are placed on agonist muscle and 2 on antagonist; parameters will be set so the current alternates between stimulating one set of electrodes and other set. • Establish correct parameters for NMES treatment. • Turn on unit and monitor patient's response. Let unit run for a few cycles before leaving patient (if you are doing so). • Make sure patient has a call bell if you are leaving patient alone. • Check patient's skin and ask for feedback after treatment.
Safety Considerations	• Monitor patient's response (verbally and visually) during treatment session. • Make sure skin prep is done before applying electrodes.
Advantages	• Patient may be able to perform therapy interventions while connected to unit • Can promote muscle strengthening or movement
Disadvantages	• Larger units are more expensive • Patient may find certain settings uncomfortable and require education or gradual increase

in the treatment and begin to feel what it is like to move the muscle themselves. Even if the voluntary contraction is minimal, it can still prove to be beneficial.

NMES can be used not only to strengthen muscles, but also to re-educate muscles injured by trauma or a neurological insult, reduce muscle guarding/spasms by fatiguing the muscle, or reduce edema by replicating a muscle pump. Table 10-6 details how to administer NMES safely, and Table 10-7 lists the NMES parameters. Figures 10-17 and 10-18 show the various types of NMES units one might encounter in the clinic.

Russian Current

Russian electrical stimulation, or Russian current, so called because of the research by Russian scientist Dr Yakov Kots[28] on Russian athletes, is considered a subset of NMES in that it does aim to strengthen the muscle, but it also has

been shown to increase muscle force.[29] Russian current is an AC that is delivered in bursts. Parameters typically follow a 10/50/10 set-up, meaning 10 muscle contractions that last for 10 seconds with 50 seconds of off time (ie, 10:50 on:off time). Duration of treatment is usually about 10 minutes (or about 10 contractions) because the muscle will fatigue rapidly. Some patients report Russian current to be uncomfortable because the contractions are strong. While the original research was conducted on healthy individuals, Russian current is often used for patients unable to generate voluntary contractions on their own with the goal of strengthening the muscle[30] or preventing atrophy.[31] In other studies, the clinicians ask the patient to perform voluntary contractions concomitant with the electrical stimulation if the patient is able. It is a point of debate among some clinicians as to whether a voluntary contraction is beneficial.

Table 10-7
Transcutaneous Electrical Nerve Stimulation Parameters

NMES Goal	pps (Pulse Frequency)[27]	Pulse Duration (μs)	Amplitude (Intensity) in mA	On:Off Times/Ratio[27]	Ramp Time[27]	Duration
Muscle strengthening	50 to 80	300 to 600	Until strong contraction	10 sec on, 30 sec off; 1:3	1 to 3 sec	10 to 20 min (10 to 20 contractions)
Muscle re-education	20 to 50	300 to 600	Until strong contraction	1:1 or 1:5, as clinician dictates	1 to 3 sec	Varies depending on functional task
Muscle guard/ spasm	20 to 50	300 to 600	Until strong contraction	1:1	1 to 3 sec	10 to 20 min (10 to 20 contractions)
Edema reduction (muscle pump)	20 to 50	300 to 600	Until strong contraction	2 to 5 sec on, 2 to 5 sec off; 1:1	1 to 3 sec	20 to 30 min, 3 to 5 times/ day

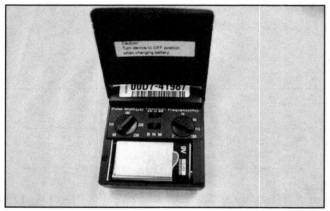

Figure 10-17. NMES unit #1.

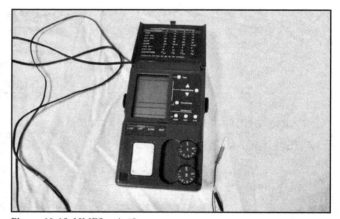

Figure 10-18. NMES unit #2.

Functional Electrical Stimulation

Functional electrical stimulation (FES) is often used for patients who require muscle reeducation. Perhaps the patient had a cerebrovascular accident (CVA), or the patient was in an accident that caused trauma to a nerve. FES is called *functional* because the electrical current is delivered in order for the patient to practice and resume a functional task. One common use is with a patient who has foot drop (or lacks dorsiflexion during the swing phase of gait); electrodes are applied to the common peroneal (fibular) nerve (in the tibialis anterior muscle) to elicit dorsiflexion during a gait training activity.[32] Similarly, electrodes may be used on the upper extremity to promote functional tasks.[33] The idea is that the patient performs as much voluntary contraction as possible while the stimulation is occurring and while performing the task requiring practice, thus re-educating the muscle. FES can be applied using a typical electrical stimulation unit; however, there are versions that patients can wear at home or in the clinic while performing specific tasks, such as Bioness units for the upper and lower extremity.[34] Some of the devices benefit from being wireless so the patient can perform the functional task unencumbered.

Patterned Electrical Neuromuscular Stimulation

Patterned electrical neuromuscular stimulation (PENS) is a relatively new type of electrical stimulation. Current delivery is based off of healthy individuals' EMG patterns during physical activity. These patterns were studied and then replicated, aiming to resemble the normal firing patterns of the muscles (agonist and antagonist).[35] Like FES,

Table 10-8

Russian, Functional Electrical Stimulation, and Patterned Electrical Neuromuscular Stimulation Parameters

NMES Goal	pps (Pulse Frequency)[29]	Pulse Duration (µs)	Amplitude (Intensity) in mA	On:Off Times/Ratio[29]	Ramp Time[29]	Duration
Russian	2500	10	Until a strong contraction is achieved, 100 mA maximum	10 sec on, 50 sec off; 1:5	1 to 2 sec	10 min
FES	20 to 50	300 to 600	Until strong contraction	1:1 or 1:5, as clinician dictates	1 to 3 sec	Varies depending on functional task
PENS	50	< 100 (70)	Until a strong contraction	Usually preset	Usually preset	Varies depending on functional task; averages 10 to 15 min

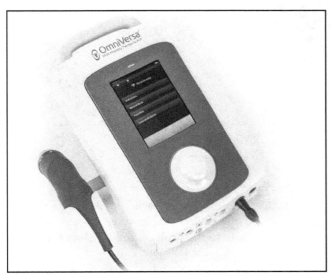

Figure 10-19. OmniStim unit.

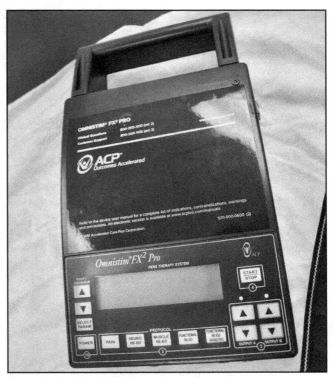

Figure 10-20. Older PENS unit.

PENS requires the patient to perform voluntary contractions in tandem with the electrical stimulation with the expectation that this combination will yield improved motor learning and performance. Unlike the discomfort some feel with Russian stimulation, PENS current is often described as comfortable. Commonly, one must use a unit specifically for the purpose of PENS treatments, such as an OmniStim device (Accelerated Care Plus; Figures 10-19 and 10-20). These units often have preset parameters for specific muscle groups. Table 10-8 provides the parameters for administering Russian, FES, and PENS treatments.

Other Types of Electrical Stimulation

So far, this section has discussed what some may consider the most commonly used or known electrical stimulation currents in the clinic. However, there are a few more to address in this chapter. Namely, this section will talk about HVPC, iontophoresis, bone growth stimulators, EMG biofeedback, and the use of electrical stimulation in combination with ultrasound.

Goal	Polarity	pps (Pulse Frequency)	Pulse Duration (µs)[36]	Amplitude (Intensity) in mA	Duration
Healing with infection present	Negative	1 to 125	5 to 200	To a comfortable tingling	30 to 60 min/day or as needed
Healing with no infection present	Positive	1 to 125	5 to 200	To a comfortable tingling	30 to 60 min as needed
Edema reduction	Negative	100	2 to 20	Strong tingling sensation	20 to 30 min

Table 10-9

High-Voltage Pulsed-Current Electrical Stimulation

Box 10-1

Research Topic

Does HVPC reduce edema? Conduct some research on this topic. Does the research differentiate between the type of injury (acute vs chronic)? How does HVPC compare to the use of NMES to create alternating muscle contractions for the reduction of edema in a limb?

High-Voltage Pulsed Current

HVPC is a type of current used primarily in the healing of wounds. It is a monophasic pulsed current that is thought to attract neutrophils, macrophages, lymphocytes, and fibroblasts to a wound bed by an electrical charge, called *galvanotaxis*.[36] HVPC uses polarity as one of its parameters, with the thought that the negative electrode (or cathode) is placed on or near the wound if it is infected and the positive electrode (anode) is placed over or near the wound if it is not infected. The other electrode is usually placed proximally to the active electrode. Some studies had the cathode always function as the active electrode, whereas others had the clinicians alternate the cathode and anode.[36]

HVPC is also thought to decrease swelling in an area by use of a polarity setting, namely, that a negative electrode (cathode) will repel the proteins in lymph fluid and decrease swelling. Alternately, some studies suggest that the current affects the permeability of microvessels, and this affects the balance of fluid and proteins in the vessels and interstitial spaces.[37] Either way, there is some evidence that HVPC can be beneficial to this goal. Table 10-9 offers the parameters for HVPC interventions. Box 10-1 provides a research topic on the use of HVPC to reduce edema.

HVPC may have some positive effects on decreasing pain, although there needs to be more research on this topic. A 2019 study showed that HVPC did decrease pain in patients with osteoarthritis, possibly thanks to its ability to decrease inflammation and the activation of the Gate Control theory, but that IFC did a more effective job of controlling pain.[38]

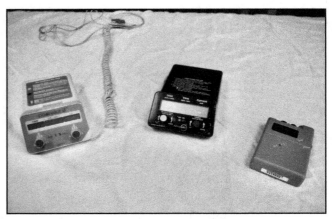

Figure 10-21. Ionto machines.

Iontophoresis

Iontophoresis uses DC to send medication directly through the skin and into the affected tissue using the polarity of the ions in the drug. Figure 10-21 shows different units used to administer iontophoresis. Using the concept that like charges repel, the ions of the drug are pushed through the skin. The benefits of iontophoresis include the ability to apply the medication directly to the tissue in question, rather than the patient taking an oral medication that must travel systemically. It also avoids the need for injections, and the dosage of the medication is easier to control. There are relatively few if any side effects as long as the patient can tolerate the drug being used.

Many different drugs can be delivered via iontophoresis, including lidocaine for pain (positively charged), dexamethasone for inflammation (negatively charged), or zinc for wounds (positively charged). One must know the drug's polarity to set the parameters correctly; whatever the polarity of the drug, the same polarity in the active electrode is used to repel the drug into the tissue. Table 10-10 lists some of the most commonly used medications and their polarities. The medication is applied to the active electrode per the amount usually found on the electrode/box, measured in milliliters. The drug is applied using a

Table 10-10
Commonly Used Medications for Iontophoresis

Medications	Indications	Polarity
Acetic acid	Calcium deposits, myositis ossificans	Negative
Calcium chloride	Scar tissue, muscle spasms	Negative
Copper sulfate	Fungal infections	Positive
Dexamethasone	Inflammation	Negative
Iodine	Scars, adhesive capsulitis	Negative
Lidocaine	Analgesia, inflammation	Positive
Magnesium sulfate	Muscle spasms, ischemia	Positive
Salicylates	Muscle/joint pain	Negative
Zinc oxide	Healing, wounds	Positive

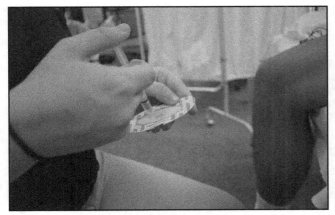

Figure 10-22. Filling electrode with syringe.

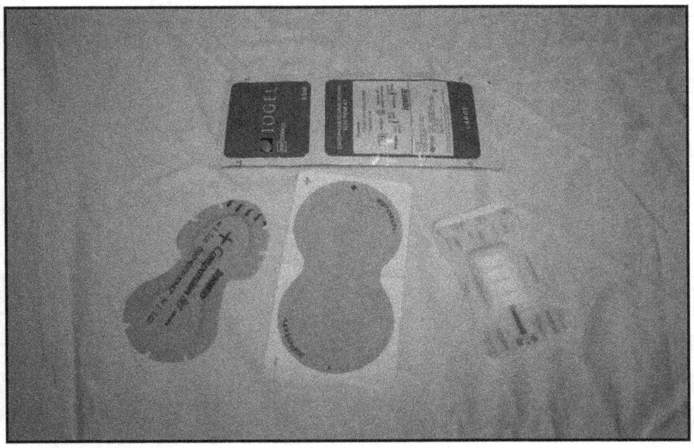

Figure 10-23. Different types of ionto electrodes.

syringe, and should fully soak the sponge area of the electrode without overfilling it (Figure 10-22). There are many different types of iontophoresis electrodes (Figure 10-23). The active electrode is then placed over or near the affected area, and a dispersive electrode should be placed at least 2 inches (5 cm) away, usually over a large muscle belly to make the treatment more comfortable. Figure 10-24 shows an iontophoresis treatment electrode configuration. The cathode is the active electrode for negative drugs, such as dexamethasone, and the anode is the active electrode if the drug is positive, like lidocaine. The amplitude can be as high as 4 mA. Most units are capped at 4 mA so you cannot make a mistake. The treatment time is dependent on the amplitude (per patient tolerance) and the total dosage, which is usually 40 mA. There are options to administer 60 mA/min and 80 mA/min dosages, and this would depend on the goals of the treatment and the size of the active electrode. Some electrodes provide information on the total dosage. The calculation to determine the duration of treatment is amplitude (in mA) × duration (in minutes) = dosage (in mA/minutes). Therefore, a patient who can

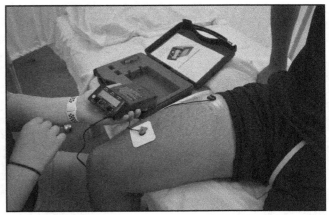

Figure 10-24. Placement of electrodes on body (over affected and dispersive).

tolerate an amplitude of 2 mA with the goal to receive a total dosage of 40 mA/min will need to receive iontophoresis for 20 minutes. If the total dosage were 80 mA/min, the duration would need to increase to 40 minutes. It is

	Table 10-11
	Procedures for Applying Iontophoresis
Equipment Needed	• Iontophoresis unit • Electrodes—active and dispersive • Wires • Medication and syringe • Alcohol wipes • Sheets, pillows • Treatment table/chair
Treatment/ Parameters	• Confirm patient does not have contraindications. • Determine optimal patient position—supine, prone, or seated. • Remove clothing and jewelry from area. • Prepare skin area before electrode placement—clean with alcohol wipe, trim excessive hair, ensure skin is intact, etc. • Withdraw medication amount per active electrode indications; apply to active electrode, being sure to saturate but not overfill electrode. • Apply active electrode over affected area; apply dispersive electrode at least 2 in (5 cm) away from the active electrode and over a muscle belly. • Establish correct parameters for iontophoresis treatment, following amplitude (in mA) × duration (in min) = dosage (in mA – min) equation. • Let unit run for a few minutes before leaving patient (if you are doing so). • Make sure patient has a call bell if you are leaving patient alone. • Check patient's skin and ask for feedback after treatment.
Safety Considerations	• Monitor patient's response (verbally and visually) during treatment session. • Make sure skin prep is done before applying electrodes. • Ensure patient is not allergic to medication being used. • Adjust amplitude, electrode size, or distance between electrodes if patient expresses discomfort.
Advantages	• Patient may be able to perform therapy interventions while receiving intervention, especially if using a battery-powered electrode • Can provide a variety of benefits depending on the drug with few side effects and no systemic absorption or need for injection
Disadvantages	• May be limited in motion if using a traditional unit • Patient may find treatment uncomfortable and require education • Patients may be allergic to drug, adhesive in electrode, or have skin reaction to treatment

important to remember this equation; some iontophoresis units calculate the time, but others do not. Table 10-11 gives details on how to administer iontophoresis, and Table 10-12 provides the parameters for iontophoresis.

There are some low-voltage patches that allow the patient to wear the patch, disconnected from a unit because it has a battery inside, for up to 24 hours while it slowly delivers the dosage of medication. Figure 10-25 shows an example of this. Many patients report that these patches are more comfortable than receiving traditional iontophoresis, which can be described as prickling by some, but the patient obviously cannot shower or get the area wet while wearing the patch.

Aside from the prickling sensation associated with iontophoresis, some safety concerns to consider are the possibility of skin irritation during or after the treatment and the possibility of burning the patient. This is because there is a build-up of charge as a result of unidirectional flow

Table 10-12
High-Voltage Pulsed-Current Electrical Stimulation

Type of Treatment	Waveform	Polarity	Amplitude	Duration
Iontophoresis	DC	Depends on drug	To patient tolerance, ≤ 4 mA	Depends on amplitude, to produce 40, 60, or 80 mA/min

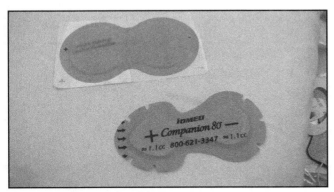

Figure 10-25. Ionto patch with battery.

Table 10-13
Ways to Make Iontophoresis More Comfortable

Lower the amplitude.
Select a larger electrode.
Move the dispersive pad farther away from active electrode.

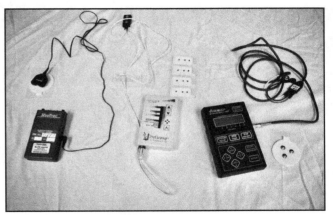

Figure 10-26. Various biofeedback units.

of charged particles, and this causes a chemical effect on the tissue under the electrode. Iontophoresis is primarily a superficial treatment, and while it is normal to observe some reddening of the skin after removing the iontophoresis electrodes, especially the active electrode, one should inspect the patient's skin for any signs of burning and take the patient's feedback seriously if they complain of discomfort. If the patient reports that the treatment is uncomfortable, the clinician can lower the amplitude, select a larger active electrode, or move the dispersive electrode farther away to make the treatment tolerable. Table 10-13 offers these reminders.

Bone Growth Stimulators

If a patient has a bone fracture that is not healing normally, the use of a bone growth stimulator might be considered. These can be noninvasive, in that the patient wears external electrodes nearly 24 hours/day, or invasive, in that the patient has a percutaneous or surgically implanted device. Invasive stimulators have mixed results with healing because the surgical nature is also affiliated with increased infections.[39] Percutaneous stimulators have a better track record.[40] These units are specifically prescribed by physicians, and the parameters are also set by the doctor.

Electromyographic Biofeedback

EMG biofeedback is different from the previously discussed electrical stimulation modalities because technically, EMG biofeedback does not provide electrical stimulation. Rather, EMG biofeedback measures the electrical activity generated by a muscle when it contracts. Specifically, an EMG biofeedback machine measures the action potentials created during a muscle contraction. Figure 10-26 shows different EMG biofeedback units.

Although EMG biofeedback does not electrically stimulate the muscles to cause a contraction, reduce edema, or heal a wound, it instead can cue a patient to either contract or relax a muscle by showing the patient what the muscle is doing. Most units have some form of lights or sound to reflect the electrical activity occurring. For example, if a patient has muscle spasms or guarding, the biofeedback unit will show the patient through increasing or different colored lights, sound, or some other means that the muscle is contracting. The therapist might then cue the patient to try to make the lights change from red to green, or to make the beeping less noisy, and the patient uses the cue from the therapist and the biofeedback unit to try to relax the muscle in question. Alternately, if the patient has a muscle they need to contract more, perhaps after having a CVA or a traumatic injury, the unit can encourage the patient by showing increasing lights and/or beeping when they are able to contract the muscle more (Figure 10-27).

Table 10-14	
Procedures for Applying Electromyographic Biofeedback	
Equipment Needed	• Biofeedback unit • Electrodes • Wires • Alcohol wipes • Sheets, pillows • Treatment table/chair
Treatment/ Parameters	• Confirm patients understand goals of treatment and what they should do. • Determine optimal patient position—supine, prone, or seated. • Remove clothing and jewelry from area. • Prepare skin area before electrode placement—clean with alcohol wipe, trim excessive hair, ensure skin is intact, etc. • Apply electrode(s) over focus area. • Establish correct parameters; if goal is muscle re-education (contraction), adjust sensitivity threshold to lowest number that picks up any action potentials in the area; if goal is muscle relaxation, adjust sensitivity threshold to pick up maximal action potentials. • If goal is muscle re-education, ask patient to contract the target muscle; you can facilitate by tapping, stroking, or having patient contract contralateral muscle. • If goal is muscle relaxation, ask patient to relax the muscle; you can facilitate this by applying heat, gentle range of motion, or promoting mental imagery or deep breathing. • As patient achieves threshold, you can adjust threshold to make it slightly more difficult for patient to achieve. • Check patient's skin and ask for feedback after treatment.
Safety Considerations	• Monitor patient's response (verbally and visually) during treatment session. • Make sure skin prep is done before applying electrodes. • Electrodes should be applied so they are parallel to muscle fibers. • Ensure patient understands goal of the session.
Advantages	• Patient is a part of treatment • Patient can be motivated by lights/audio and make changes
Disadvantages	• Patient may not understand goal or how to participate • Setting parameters on unit can be difficult for clinician

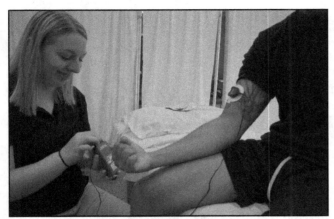

Figure 10-27. Use of EMG biofeedback for strengthening.

In this way, EMG biofeedback can be said that it could decrease pain, in that it incites the patient to relax spasming muscles, or that it can increase function by providing motivation for the patient to make the muscle contract. There are drawbacks to using EMG biofeedback, however. While there is little likelihood of injuring the patient—as there could be with traditional electrical stimulation—and there are also few real contraindications, EMG biofeedback can be difficult to use. The clinician needs to be familiar with the unit and how to set the parameters. Table 10-14 provides details on the application of EMG biofeedback; parameter options are specific to the unit being used. Most units at least allow for a sensitivity setting; the higher the sensitivity, the more action potentials detected. Therefore, high sensitivity settings should be used when attempting muscle relaxation, and lower sensitivity should be used when the goal is muscle re-education.

Another potential drawback is that the patient needs to have buy-in to the treatment; patients need to be well educated on how the unit works and what the goal of the treatment is, as well as their role in the treatment. Patients are actively relaxing or contracting the muscle or body part in question, and they need to understand that before embarking on the treatment session.

Ultrasound/Electrical Stimulation Combination

Chapter 4 briefly mentioned that one can combine ultrasound and electrical stimulation into the same treatment, often referred to as *combo*. Merging ultrasound with electrical stimulation is useful because it combines the benefits of ultrasound with those of electrical stimulation, although more recent research questions the overall efficacy of using this type of treatment. Because ultrasound is one of the few modalities shown to penetrate up to 5 cm, one could potentially target deeper tissues with a combo setting; therefore, one would likely select 3 MHz to accomplish this goal. One must, of course, be mindful of the contraindications of both modalities before application.

One must have a unit that allows for combination treatments; in this case, the ultrasound head serves as one electrode while another actual electrode is placed on the patient's body. The ultrasound head will deliver both acoustic and electrical energy. The same rules of application for ultrasound apply, in that gel or lotion must be used, and the sound head must continuously move at the recommended speed of 4 cm/s. When the head passes over the muscle motor point, one may see a muscle contraction. The ultrasound can also increase tissue temperature. Combo treatments are often used for muscle guarding or trigger points, but any indication for ultrasound or electrical stimulation is applicable. Parameters are individually set on the unit (usually one first sets the ultrasound parameters followed by the electrical stimulation parameters), and they should follow the guidelines set out for the specific therapeutic intention. Figure 10-28 shows a patient receiving an ultrasound/electrical stimulation combo.

SAFETY CONCERNS

There are a few safety considerations when using electricity, the most obvious being the risk of electrocution. All units should be checked annually to ensure they are functioning correctly. Electrical devices should be properly grounded to avoid the risk of electrocution, and patients should be educated to not use take-home devices when in the shower, bath, or any time there is a risk of getting the device and electrodes wet.

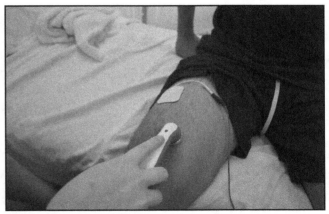

Figure 10-28. Patient receiving (set-up for) combo.

Electrical currents administered to the skin can cause burns. The risk for burns may increase depending on the type of current being used or the method and set-up of the intervention. It is important that the clinician takes care to prepare the patient's tissue correctly for treatment and to monitor the patient's skin before, during, and after the intervention to ensure no burning has occurred. Certain steps, such as ensuring the wires are not frayed, the electrodes adhere fully to the skin, the electrodes are larger, or the electrodes are far enough apart, can prevent burns. Electrodes can be used more than once, but they should be replaced regularly or any time the adhesive becomes ineffective.

Skin preparation can ensure proper adherence of the electrodes, thus reducing the risk of burns. The skin should be wiped clean and dry with either a damp washcloth or the use of alcohol preparation pads, especially if the patient has applied lotion to the area. If the skin area has excess hair, the hair should be trimmed, but not shaved. Shaving creates microtears in the tissue, which could allow uneven distribution of the current into the tissue, causing discomfort and possible burns.

In addition, electrode placement can prevent burning. Electrodes that are too small or placed close to each other may result in burns or discomfort because the current travels more superficially; larger electrodes placed farther apart will be safer and more comfortable.

Electrode placement is important for other reasons. Avoid placing electrodes over the carotid artery (as mentioned in the contraindications section), the eyes, the gonads, the chest areas over the heart (whether or not the patient has a pacemaker), and not internally unless the device is designed specifically for that treatment.[19] Electrodes also should not be placed over bony prominences. Electrode placement is also important to consider depending on the treatment. If treating a wound, for example, the active electrode should be on or very close to the wound, or the 2 electrodes can surround it. During an IFC treatment, one must use 4 electrodes that surround the area and crisscross to achieve the interference of the 2 currents. The clinician should make sure to document specifically where electrodes are placed during the treatment to ensure the ability of replication.

When turning on the electrical stimulation, the clinician should be sure to go slowly to carefully monitor the patient's response. One might be looking for a tetanic contraction of the muscle, but one should monitor that the patient is tolerating this setting well. If the unit has an AC (or an on:off time), make sure to turn up the intensity only during the "on" time. Otherwise, one could surprise the patient when the on time begins and one has unwittingly increased the intensity too much.

DOCUMENTATION

When applying electrical stimulation, there are certain parameters that should be documented. As with other treatments, be sure to document the patient's position, the area being treated, and the goal of the treatment. The parameters of the specific treatment should be specified, as well as the location of the electrodes. If one had to adjust the parameters during the session, indicate what and how they were adjusted. Include the duration of the treatment and the patient's response (either verbally or physically) to the treatment. Below are a few examples of a case scenario and documentation.

Diagnosis: Patient is in therapy seeing wound care team for a chronic venous stasis ulcer on the right lateral ankle.

O: Patient supine with right lower extremity elevated on 2 pillows. Patient's skin cleaned with alcohol wipe before treatment. Received HVPC electrical stimulation to the right lower extremity × 45 minutes with negative electrode placed over the wound and positive electrode place proximally on the right gastrocnemius. Frequency set at 100 pps, negative polarity, intensity to tingling sensation at 2 mA. Patient reported no discomfort during the session and skin inspected after treatment.

Diagnosis: Patient in therapy after having right middle cerebral artery stroke status post 6 weeks ago.

O: Receiving FES to the left tibialis anterior to promote dorsiflexion during swing phase of gait. Applied 2 electrodes over the left tibialis anterior superiorly and inferiorly. Parameters set at 35 pps, 300 μs, 1:2 ratio to account for gait speed on a 1-second ramp, amplitude at 3.5 mA to produce strong contraction. Patient encouraged to produce contraction on his own. Received stimulation while ambulating on treadmill × 10 minutes because of patient fatigue. Patient reported no discomfort during the treatment but reported muscle felt fatigued after session completed.

CONCLUSION

Electrical stimulation is a term that encompasses a wide assortment of settings and goals. One can strengthen or re-educate a muscle, reduce edema, decrease pain, heal a wound, or help a bone grow. For electrical stimulation to be a skilled intervention, the clinician should understand how the nerves, muscles, and tissues are affected by electrical current, as well as how the parameters can be modified to achieve the goal set forth by the supervising physical therapist. While there are some important contraindications to consider, as well as safety concerns that surround the use of electricity, many studies support the use of electricity to address these various concerns.

REVIEW QUESTIONS

1. What are the 3 types of electrical current? What do these designations mean?
2. List the contraindications for using electrical stimulation.
3. Describe how a muscle contraction occurs physiologically.
4. Discuss the difference among conventional, acupuncture, and burst TENS.
5. What are the benefits of using IFC vs TENS for pain relief?
6. What are the indications for using electrical stimulation to produce muscle contractions?
7. How does EMG biofeedback work? Would you set the unit as more or less sensitive if the goal is to re-educate a muscle? Explain.
8. What are the benefits of administering iontophoresis to a patient? What type of current does iontophoresis use?
9. Why would one want to use electrical stimulation in combination with ultrasound? What benefits does such a treatment yield?
10. List at least 3 safety concerns one must be aware of before or during treatment with electrical stimulation.
11. You have a patient receiving dexamethasone administered via iontophoresis to the plantar aspect of the foot for plantar fasciitis. What polarity is dexamethasone and what polarity would you select for your active electrode? If the patient can tolerate an amplitude of 3 mA with the goal of achieving a dosage of 60 mA/min, how many minutes must the patient receive treatment?
12. You are seeing your patient for upper trapezius pain secondary to a fall, and you want to use electrical stimulation to help decrease the pain. The pain covers a large area. What pain reduction electrical stimulation setting/modality would you select? Why? What would be your parameters? How would you document this in your "O" section?

13. Your patient sprained her right ankle yesterday and presents today with significant pain and swelling. What electrical stimulation modality/setting would be most beneficial to help with this patient's swelling? What parameters would you set? How would you document this in your "O" section?

CASE STUDY 1

Your patient is a 68-year-old woman who had a right CVA (left side affected) with weakness in her left lower extremity, specifically her anterior tibialis. She is unable to dorsiflex fully and, therefore, needs the use of an ankle foot orthosis during ambulation, as well as the use of a hemi-walker. The goal is to use electrical stimulation to strengthen the anterior tibialis to promote improved dorsiflexion and normal gait.
1. What tissues are injured?
2. What electrical stimulation technique would you use for this patient? Why?
3. What parameters would you use for this patient?
4. What are the contraindications for this treatment?
5. What other therapeutic intervention(s) would you use for this patient? Why?

CASE STUDY 2

A 49-year-old man is in therapy after sustaining a motor vehicle accident in which his left ankle was crushed. He had surgery with pins and screws placed and was in a cast for 12 weeks. Now that the cast has been removed, he is complaining of pain, 5 to 7/10, with the pain worse when attempting ambulation or prolonged standing. He also has some swelling and tenderness in the area and prefers to not wear a sock or shoe on that foot. The physician reports that everything has healed properly. Your supervising physical therapist wants you to perform electrical stimulation for this patient to reduce pain to restore function.
1. What tissues are affected?
2. What phase of healing is this patient in?
3. What electrical stimulation technique would you use for this patient? Why?
4. What are the parameters you would use?
5. What other therapeutic intervention(s) would you recommend for this patient? Why?

REFERENCES

1. Holmes R. *The Age of Wonder: The Romantic Generation and the Discovery of the Beauty and Terror of Science.* Vintage Books (Random House); 2010.
2. Ashrafi M, Alonso-Rasgado T, Baguneid M, Bayat A. The efficacy of electrical stimulation in lower extremity cutaneous wound healing: a systematic review. *Exp Dermatol.* 2017;26(2):171-178.
3. Gardner SE, Frantz RA, Schmidt FL. Effect of electrical stimulation on chronic wound healing: a meta-analysis. *Wound Repair Regen.* 1999;7(6):495-503.
4. Khouri C, Kotzki S, Roustit M, Blaise S, Gueyffier F, Cracowski J. Hierarchical evaluation of electrical stimulation protocols for chronic wound healing: an effect size meta-analysis. *Wound Repair Regen.* 2017;25(5):883-891.
5. Reza Asadi M, Torkaman G, Hedayati M, Mofid M. Role of sensory and motor intensity of electrical stimulation on fibroblastic growth factor-2 expression, inflammation, vascularization, and mechanical strength of full-thickness wounds. *J Rehabil Res Dev.* 2013;50(4):489-498.
6. Lallyett C, Yeung CY, Nielson RH, et al. Changes in S100 proteins identified in healthy skin following electrical stimulation: relevance for wound healing. *Adv Skin Wound Care.* 2018;31(7):322-327.
7. Feger MA, Goetschius J, Love H, Saliba SA, Hertel J. Electrical stimulation as a treatment intervention to improve function, edema or pain following acute lateral ankle sprains: a systematic review. *Phys Ther Sport.* 2015;16(4):361-369.
8. Kadı MR, Hepgüler S, Atamaz FC, et al. Is interferential current effective in the management of pain, range of motion, and edema following total knee arthroplasty surgery? A randomized double-blind controlled trial. *Clin Rehabil.* 2019;33(6):1027-1034.
9. Burgess LC, Immins T, Swain I, Wainwright TW. Effectiveness of neuromuscular electrical stimulation for reducing oedema: a systematic review. *J Rehabil Med.* 2019;51(4):237-243.
10. Sandoval MC, Ramirez CR, Camargo DM, Russo TL, Salvini TF. Effect of high-voltage electrical stimulation on the albumin and histamine serum concentrations, edema, and pain in acute joint inflammation of rats. *Braz J Phys Ther.* 2015;19(2):89-96.
11. Snyder AR, Perotti AL, Lam KC, Bay RC. The influence of high-voltage electrical stimulation on edema formation after acute injury: a systematic review. *J Sport Rehabil.* 2010;19(4):436-451.
12. Bhavsar MB, Han Z, DeCoster T, Leppik L, Oliveira KMC, Barker J. Electrical stimulation-based bone fracture treatment, if it works so well why do not more surgeons use it? *Eur J Trauma Emerg Surg.* 2019;46(2):245-264.
13. Martinez-Rondanelli A, Martinez JP, Moncada M, Manzi E, Pinedo CR, Cadavid H. Electromagnetic stimulation as coadjuvant in the healing of diaphyseal femoral fractures: a randomized controlled trial. *Columb Med (Cali).* 2014;45(2):67-71.

14. Carlson BM. The biology of long-term denervated skeletal muscle. *Eur J Transl Myol*. 2014;24(1):3293.

15. Gordon T. Electrical stimulation to enhance axon regeneration after peripheral nerve injuries in animal models and humans. *Neurotherapeutics*. 2016;13(2):295-310.

16. Chandrasekaran S, Davis J, Bersch I, Goldberg G, Gorgey AS. Electrical stimulation and denervated muscles after spinal cord injury. *Neural Regen Res*. 2020;15(8):1397-1407.

17. Srivastava N, Joshi S. Comparison between effectiveness of iontophoresis and conventional therapy in the management of plantar fasciitis. *Indian J Physiother Occup Ther*. 2017;11(1):1-5.

18. Bergeron-Vézina K, Corriveau H, Martel M, Harvey MP, Léonard G. High- and low-frequency transcutaneous electrical nerve stimulation does not reduce experimental pain in elderly individuals. *Pain*. 2015;156(10):2093-2099.

19. Johnson M. Transcutaneous electrical nerve stimulation: mechanisms, clinical application and evidence. *Rev Pain*. 2007;1(1):7-11.

20. Watson T. Transcutaneous electrical nerve stimulation. Electrotherapy on the web. Published 2020. Accessed June 11, 2020. http://www.electrotherapy.org/m/modality/transcutaneous-electrical-nerve-stimulation-tens#Mechanism%20of%20Action

21. Watson T. Interferential therapy. Electrotherapy on the web. Published 2020. Accessed June 14, 2020. http://www.electrotherapy.org/modality/interferential-therapy

22. US National Library of Medicine. Acute effects of interferential current on edema, pain, and muscle strength in patient with distal radius fracture. Published February 26, 2018. Accessed June 14, 2020. https://clinicaltrials.gov/ct2/show/study/NCT03438864

23. Ariel E. Penetration depth of therapeutic electrical currents in various electrodes locations and different current components in chronic low back pain patients. *Physiotherapy*. 2015;101(1):E83-E84.

24. Demirtürk F, Akbayrak T, Karakaya IC, et al. Interferential current versus biofeedback results in urinary stress incontinence. *Swiss Med Wkly*. 2008;138(21-22):317-321.

25. Delitto A, Snyder-Mackler L. Augmentation using percutaneous electrical stimulation. *Phys Ther*. 1990;70(3):158-164.

26. Reidel LT, Cecchele B, Sachetti A, Calegari L. Effects of neuromuscular electrostimulation of quadriceps on the functionality of fragile and pre-frail hospitalized older adults: randomized clinical trial. *Fisioterapia e Pesquisa*. 2020;27(2):126-132.

27. Doucet BM, Lam A, Griffin L. Neuromuscular electrical stimulation for skeletal muscle function. *Yale J Biol Med*. 2012;85(2):201-215.

28. Ward AR, Shkuratova N. Russian electrical stimulation: the early experiments. *Phys Ther*. 2002;82(10):1019-1030.

29. Watson T. Russian stimulation and burst mode alternating current (BMAC). Published 2020. Accessed June 19, 2020. http://www.electrotherapy.org/modality/russian-stimulation-and-burst-mode-alternating-current-bmac-

30. Heggannavar A, Sharmayat S, Nerurkar S, AKamble S. Effect of Russian current on quadriceps muscle strength in subjects with primary osteoarthritis of knee: a randomized control trial. *Int J Physiother Res*. 2014;2(3):555-560.

31. de Souza Bueno CR, Pereira M, Favaretto Jr IA, et al. Electrical stimulation attenuates morphological alterations and prevents atrophy of the denervated cranial tibial muscle. *Einstein (Sao Paulo)*. 2017;15(1):71-76.

32. Bulley C, Mercer TH, Hooper JE, Cowan P, Scott S, van der Linden ML. Experiences of functional electrical stimulation (FES) and ankle foot orthoses (AFOs) for foot-drop in people with multiple sclerosis. *Disabil Rehabil Assist Technol*. 2014;10(6):458-467.

33. Kawashima N, Popovic MR, Zivanovic V. Effect of intensive functional electrical stimulation therapy on upper-limb motor recovery after stroke: case study of a patient with chronic stroke. *Physiother Can*. 2013;65(1):20-28.

34. Bioness. Our products. Published 2020. Accessed June 21, 2020. http://www.bioness.com/Products.php

35. Gulick DT, Castel JC, Palermo FX, Draper DO. Effect of patterned electrical neuromuscular stimulation on vertical jump in collegiate athletes. *Sports Health*. 2011;3(2):152-157.

36. Polak A, Franek A, Taradaj J. High-voltage pulsed current electrical stimulation in wound treatment. *Adv Wound Care (New Rochelle)*. 2014;3(2):104-117.

37. Mendel FC, Caputi CD, Karnes JL, Fish DR. High voltage pulsed current using surface electrodes: effect on acute edema formation after hyperflexion injury in frogs. *J Orthop Sports Phys Ther*. 1992;16(3):140-144.

38. Singh SK, Agrawa R, Akbani R. Comparison of the effect of high voltage pulsed current v/s interferential therapy on pain and WOMAC in patients with knee osteoarthritis. *Indian J Physiother Occup Ther*. 2019;13(4):112-116.

39. Hughes MS, Anglen JO. The use of implantable bone stimulators in nonunion treatment. *Orthopedics*. 2010;33(3):151.

40. Yang BY, Huang TC, Chen YS, Yao CH. Reconstructive effects of percutaneous electrical stimulation combined with GGT composite on large bone defect in rats. *Evid Based Complement Alternat Med*. 2013;2013:607201.

Unit VI

Electromagnetic Agents

Chapter 11

Shortwave Diathermy

KEY TERMS Capacitance | Continuous | Inductance | Pulsed

KEY ABBREVIATIONS PSWD | SWD

CHAPTER OBJECTIVES

1. Discuss what shortwave diathermy is and its different techniques.
2. Explain the physiological effects of shortwave diathermy, including the difference between capacitance and inductance techniques.
3. Understand the guidelines and considerations for the application of shortwave diathermy as a physical therapy intervention.
4. Explain the indications and contraindications for shortwave diathermy interventions.
5. Demonstrate adherence to safety when applying shortwave diathermy.
6. Compare the difference between continuous and pulsed settings in shortwave diathermy.
7. Apply knowledge of diathermy set-up and parameters to case scenarios.
8. Document shortwave diathermy interventions correctly in a patient's chart.

INTRODUCTION

Diathermy is an electromagnetic modality that is typically used to create heat in the body's tissues. Like ultrasound, diathermy has a nonthermal setting that can be used for specific interventions. While diathermy can be either shortwave or microwave, this chapter will focus primarily on shortwave diathermy (SWD). Figure 11-1 shows a diathermy unit. Diathermy is currently coming back as a modality used in the clinic; it went through a period during which it was not frequently used or even taught in physical therapist assistant programs. More recently, research has indicated that SWD can provide effective and deeper heating of tissues, as well as possibly promote healing.[1-3] As a result, clinics have begun using diathermy and programs have resumed teaching diathermy. SWD has been shown to penetrate between 3 and 6 cm, so it is comparable to ultrasound in that it can be beneficial to treat deeper tissues.[4]

PHYSIOLOGICAL EFFECTS OF SHORTWAVE DIATHERMY

SWD can have thermal or nonthermal effects, depending on the parameters set on the unit. The type of electrodes used for thermal effects, which are either capacitive, or dielectric, electrodes or inductive electrodes, determine whether the thermal effects are more superficial or deep.

Thermal Effects

Diathermy is primarily used to generate heat in tissues, so it makes sense that this is the main physiological effect.

Memolo J.
Therapeutic Agents for the Physical Therapist Assistant
(pp 141-147). © 2022 SLACK Incorporated.

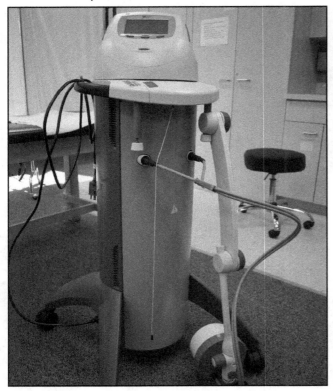

Figure 11-1. SWD unit.

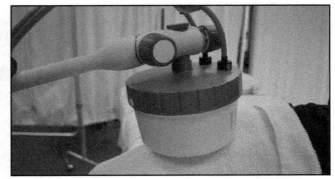

Figure 11-2. SWD unit with drum positioned over tissue.

Inductive Electrodes

Inductive diathermy creates a high-frequency current via a coil that generates a rapidly reversing magnetic field. This coil is inside a drum attached to an adjustable arm, and the drum should be directly over the body part being treated (Figure 11-2). The reversing magnetic field creates eddy currents and electric fields, which in turn create heat.[5] The heating is deeper with this type of treatment.

Nonthermal Effects

While both continuous and pulsed SWD can generate heat, pulsed SWD is also known for its nonthermal effects on the tissue. Namely, pulsed SWD has been shown to have positive effects on fibroblast and chondrocyte proliferation, indicating that it may be beneficial to promote healing in soft tissues, including wounds.[3] The research on this potential effect of SWD, however, is limited, and more recent studies would be beneficial to support this claim.[6]

INDICATIONS AND CONTRAINDICATIONS OF SHORTWAVE DIATHERMY

As mentioned previously, SWD has indications similar to those of any thermal modality. These include pain, decreased ROM, muscle guarding or muscle spasm, decreased blood flow, or soft-tissue injuries and possibly wounds. Box 11-1 provides an opportunity for further research on the use of SWD.

Contraindications should also sound familiar. Pacemakers are on the list because the electrical currents could disrupt the function of the pacemaker. Pregnancy is also at the top of the list because of the potential adverse effects on the fetus. If the patient is currently hemorrhaging, continuous SWD is contraindicated. Pulsed SWD can also generate heat, which could exacerbate bleeding, so it should be considered a precaution for treatment. Other contraindications include treating the low back or abdomen of women during menstruation, over the abdomen of women with an intrauterine device, or over metal unless the dosage is very low. Cancer, especially in the area being

The results of tissue heating are similar to those of any heating modality: increased circulation, increased range of motion (ROM), stimulated tissue healing, and reduced pain. It has been shown that both continuous and pulsed SWD can generate heat, and that tissue temperature can increase by as much as 3°C. Because diathermy's heat can penetrate deeper tissues, it can be an appealing modality over other thermal modalities. Although it can penetrate as deeply as ultrasound, diathermy has the added benefit of also addressing larger areas of the body. How does SWD generate heat? This has something to do with the type of electrodes used in an SWD treatment. These are classified as either capacitive/dielectric or inductive electrodes.

Capacitive/Dielectric Electrodes

When the capacitance type of diathermy is used, there is an alternating voltage generated between 2 electrodes that creates an alternating electric field.[5] The electrodes are placed on either side of the body part so that the electrical field penetrates that part of the body, therefore making the patient a part of the electrical circuit. The molecules in the tissue try to align with the changing electric field, and this rapid movement of molecules produces heat in the tissues.[5] These electrodes are most often 2 metal plates enclosed in plastic.[5] The heating is more superficial with this treatment.

Table 11-1

Indications, Contraindications, and Physiological Effects of Shortwave Diathermy

Indications	Contraindications	Physiological Effects
Decreased blood flow	Pacemaker	Alternating electric field, creates molecular movement and heat
Decreased ROM	Pregnancy	Rapidly reversing magnetic field, creates eddy currents and heat
Muscle guarding/spasms	Deep vein thrombosis	Fibroblast and chondrocyte proliferation (nonthermal)
Soft-tissue/wound healing	Over active hemorrhage	Increased collagen extensibility
Pain reduction	Over abdomen of women when menstruating	Increased metabolic rate
	Over intrauterine device	Pain reduction (gate control)
	Over eyes	Increased local tissue temperature
	Over gonads	Vasodilation
	Over metal (internal or external)	
	Over epiphyseal plates (precaution)	
	Cancer (precaution)	
	Impaired cognition/sensation (precaution)	

treated, is at least a precaution, because diathermy could promote metastasis of the cancer. For similar reasons, one should not administer diathermy over an area of active infection. One should not treat a patient with continuous SWD if the patient has acute injuries or inflammation; pulsed SWD would be more appropriate until the injury is classified as subacute or chronic. As with most modalities, diathermy should not be administered over the eyes or reproductive organs. As always, never perform diathermy on a patient who has a thrombus or thrombophlebitis. Precautions include over the epiphyseal plates of children, as we do not know the effects that it might have on growth, as well as treating patients with reduced sensation or cognition. Table 11-1 lists the indications, contraindications, and physiological effects of SWD.

APPLICATION METHODS

Diathermy settings typically include whether the duty cycle is continuous or pulsed, the duration, the intensity, and the patient positioning. Some units provide preset dosages categorized as dose I, II, III, and IV, with I being little to no perception of heat, II being slight heating, III being a pleasant or comfortable heating, and IV being a strong but tolerable heating.[7] Figure 11-3 provides an example of these dosage options on a diathermy unit. Most units also allow for manual settings of the parameters, which we will discuss here.

Similar to ultrasound, SWD can be divided into continuous or pulsed treatment settings. These terms are sometimes used interchangeably with the aforementioned thermal and nonthermal settings of diathermy, as continuous SWD generates heat and pulsed SWD generates less heat or no heat.

Continuous SWD is when the machine is on 100% of the time and the unit is generating either the alternating electric field or magnetic current all the time. There is no on or off time and, therefore, the patient should feel heat from the machine during the treatment. Ideally, the heat is comfortable, although some settings may describe the heat sensation as "vigorous." Continuous diathermy is the setting of choice when one wants to heat up tissues and yield the physiological effects of heat: vasodilation, decrease of

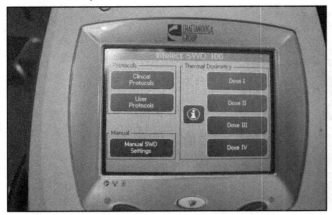

Figure 11-3. Screenshot of Chattanooga dosages.

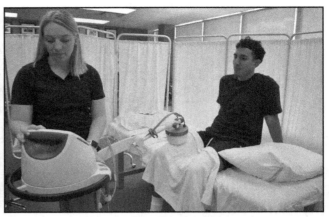

Figure 11-4. Towel between electrode and tissue.

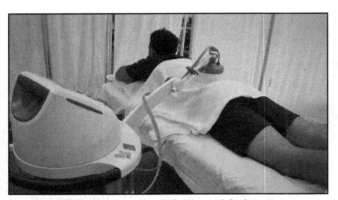

Figure 11-5. Patient positioned with draping and diathermy.

pain via Gate Control theory, and increased ROM or tissue extensibility. As with other thermal modalities, continuous SWD should not be used for acute injuries.

Pulsed SWD, alternately, does have an on/off setting, meaning that the output is on at consistent intervals or pulses. The off time is often longer than the on time, so although the settings allow heat to be generated, the longer off time allows for the heat to dissipate. This means that a patient receiving pulsed SWD may report the sensation of heat and the tissue may increase in temperature, but it is just as likely that the patient will report no heating sensation at all. Just as a continuous setting correlates to thermal effects, pulsed SWD correlates to the nonthermal effects discussed earlier. In some units, the "on" time of a pulse is also referred to as the *pulse duration* or *pulse width* and is measured as microseconds (μsec). These terms will vary depending on the unit being used. Pulsed SWD can be used both for acute and chronic injuries and can decrease pain and promote soft-tissue healing.

Just as with other modalities, SWD has additional parameters to adjust depending on the goals of the treatment. One thing to consider is the patient position. Positioning is an important factor of treating the patient and as a part of the documentation. With regard to SWD, consider whether the unit has capacitive or inductive plates.

Recall that capacitive plates make the patient a part of the electrical circuit, so the body part should be placed between the 2 plates. The space between the plates and the body part should be the same on both sides. Inductive plates do not make the patient a part of the circuit, and these are often in the form of a drum electrode. In this case, the drum should be close to the skin but not in direct contact, and the therapist should place a towel between the drum and the skin to absorb moisture, as the accumulation of sweat droplets could create hot spots on the tissue. Figure 11-4 shows a setup using a towel for sweat absorption. The patient should otherwise be placed in a position of comfort with proper draping for modesty and comfort (Figure 11-5).

Once the patient is positioned correctly and the electrodes are in the right place, and after the decision has been made whether to use continuous or pulsed SWD, there are a few other settings to adjust. One is the intensity, on some units called the *power* or *output*. This is often measured in units of watts (W), and maxes out at a certain number on some machines. Another parameter is the pulse rate, sometimes measured in hertz (Hz). This represents the number of pulses delivered per second, and there is not much evidence that specific numbers yield specific outcomes, although this combined with the pulse rate can affect the overall output of the machine, which is important.[8] Pulse duration (width) and pulse rate are parameters set only when pulsed SWD is selected; when applying continuous SWD, only intensity (output or power) and duration of treatment are parameters one can set.

The final parameter is the duration of treatment, which varies depending on whether one is applying continuous or pulsed SWD. Typically, if one is administering continuous SWD, the duration is up to about 20 minutes; when applying pulsed SWD, treatment time can be increased to about 30 minutes, but it is difficult to find recommendations to exceed that duration. Figure 11-6 shows the various settings one can adjust. Table 11-2 lists all the steps to applying diathermy.

	Table 11-2
	Procedures for Applying Shortwave Diathermy
Equipment Needed	• Diathermy unit • Alcohol wipes • Towel • Sheets, pillows • Treatment table/chair
Treatment/ Parameters	• Confirm patient does not have contraindications to treatment. • Determine optimal patient position—supine, prone, or seated—as well as position of diathermy electrode(s). • Remove clothing and jewelry from area. • Prepare skin area before treatment—clean and wipe dry area. • Set up plates according to whether they are capacitive or inductive. Capacitive are placed on either side of the body part equally distanced. Inductive are placed close or in contact with tissue, usually with a towel over treatment area to absorb sweat. • Establish correct parameters, including pulsed or continuous setting, pulse rate and duration if using pulsed SWD, and power/output and treatment duration. Alternatively, select dose I, II, III, or IV if your unit uses these parameters. • Explain to the patient what to expect to feel during treatment (more heat for continuous, possibly little to no heat with pulsed). • Begin treatment. • Provide patient with a call light/button/bell if you plan to leave patient unattended. • Check patient's skin and ask for feedback after treatment.
Safety Considerations	• Monitor patient's response (verbally and visually) during treatment session. • Make sure skin preparation is done before starting treatment. • Place signs around area and have patient in secluded area to prevent injury to others. • Make sure you have a towel between electrode and tissue to prevent burning.
Advantages	• Treatment is typically comfortable for patient
Disadvantages	• Parameters can vary depending on unit • Risk of burning patient • Patient has to remain relatively still during treatment session

Safety Concerns

The primary adverse effects of SWD are burns, so the therapist should take care to prevent these from occurring. If dosages are excessively high or if certain tissues such as fat are receiving the treatment, the risk of burns increases. Sweating, which is likely during continuous SWD, also increases the risk of burning, which is why the therapist should clean and thoroughly dry the skin receiving the treatment and why using a towel between the electrode and the tissue is recommended.

Awareness and avoidance of the listed contraindications is another important safety factor. Ideally, SWD is administered in its own room or space in the clinic. Often, for those who are pregnant or those with pacemakers,

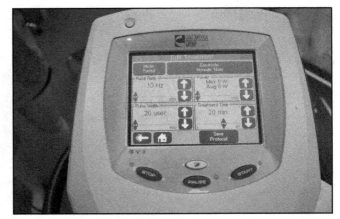

Figure 11-6. Manual settings on SWD.

therapists will place a "do not enter" sign on the door or entryway to that treatment space when the diathermy unit is on; this will help avoid accidentally causing injury not only to the patient receiving the treatment, but also to those in the adjacent area. Additionally, metal in the area of treatment may overheat; one should read the manufacturer or product materials about the rules regarding having metal in the proximity before treatment.

DOCUMENTATION

When documenting a diathermy treatment, include all parameters set, including whether the treatment was continuous or pulsed, the pulse rate and duration, if applicable, and the power/output and treatment duration. Also include the type of diathermy used (capacitive or inductive) as well as the patient and electrode positioning so the treatment could be replicated correctly the next time. Be sure to record the patient's response to the treatment. The following examples show how to document a diathermy treatment.

Diagnosis: Patient is in therapy with left low back pain rated 8/10 with activity after attempting to lift a heavy box yesterday.

O: Applied pulsed SWD using capacitive drum to patient's left lower back while patient in prone × 20 minutes. Power/output set at 150 W, drum 2 inches (5 cm) from patient with towel between drum and patient tissue, with pulse rate set at 100 µsec and pulse duration at 200 Hz. Patient reported some sensation of heat during treatment session with pain reported as 6/10 after initial session.

Diagnosis: Patient in therapy for chronic pain and decreased ROM in right ankle status post-sprain 2 weeks ago.

O: Patient received continuous SWD using capacitive drum to right lateral ankle × 15 minutes while patient in supine with right ankle elevated. Before treatment, pain reported as 6/10. Towel placed between tissue and drum, which was 1.5 inches (3.8 cm) from tissue. Power/output set at 120 W, with patient reporting comfortable but intense heating during session. After session, therapist worked on stretching the tissue to promote improved dorsiflexion and plantarflexion with less pain. Patient reported pain as 3/10 after treatment.

CONCLUSION

SWD uses electromagnetic energy to affect a person's tissues. It is helpful for diagnoses of pain, soft-tissue shortening, and soft-tissue injuries or wounds. Like ultrasound, effects can be thermal or nonthermal, as determined by the use of continuous or pulsed output. Contraindications include those for the patient, such as pacemakers, pregnancy, cancer, and blood clots, but the electromagnetic currents can affect those with pacemakers and pregnancies even if they are not receiving the treatment but are nearby. Although diathermy fell out of favor for a time, it has gained interest in the recent years. However, more studies could be conducted to support specific parameter settings and indications for use.

REVIEW QUESTIONS

1. What are the physiological effects of thermal and non-thermal diathermy?
2. Discuss the difference between capacitive and inductive plates/electrodes.
3. What are the primary parameters for SWD? How does one select or adjust these parameters?
4. List 3 contraindications and 2 precautions for the use of SWD.
5. What are some safety concerns when applying SWD to your patient?
6. Why might one select SWD over a moist hot pack to treat a patient's pain? Why would one select SWD over ultrasound?
7. You have a patient who has a right lateral ankle wound due to venous insufficiency. The wound has not been responding to traditional wound care so the physical therapist would like you to try SWD. What parameters would you select for this treatment? How would you document your "O" section?
8. Your patient had knee replacement surgery on the left knee 4 weeks ago, but she is struggling to meet the ROM requirements to be safely discharged from physical therapy. Your physical therapist would like you to try diathermy to assist with stretching. What parameters would you recommend? How would you document this treatment in your "O" section?

CASE STUDY 1

Your patient is a 79-year-old man who has osteoarthritis in his hips, with the left more painful than the right. He ambulates using a single-point cane on the right, but in the last few weeks, has been using a front-wheeled walker because of the increase in pain, rated at 8/10 at its worst. He likes to walk in the mall with his spouse for exercise 3 times/week and would like to resume walking with the single-point cane as soon as possible. Your goal is to decrease his pain to improve ambulation.

1. What tissues are affected?
2. What SWD parameters would you select for this patient? Why?
3. What are the contraindications for SWD?
4. What is another therapeutic intervention you might recommend for this patient? Why?

CASE STUDY 2

A 17-year-old woman is being seen by therapy after sustaining a patellar dislocation while playing soccer 48 hours ago. She reports the area is swollen, tender with palpation, and that ambulation on that side is painful, rated at a 5/10. She would like to return to playing soccer as soon as possible. Your goal is to decrease pain and promote healing so she can resume her sport.

1. What tissues are affected/injured?
2. What SWD parameters would you select for this patient? Why?
3. What are the physiological effects of SWD?
4. What is another therapeutic intervention you would recommend for this patient? Why?

REFERENCES

1. Marotta N, Demeco A, Inzitari MT, Caruso MG, Ammendolia A. Neuromuscular electrical stimulation and shortwave diathermy in unrecovered Bell palsy: a randomized controlled study. *Medicine (Baltimore)*. 2020;99(8):e19152.

2. Babaei-Ghazani A, Shahrami B, Fallah E, Ahadi T, Forough B, Ebadi S. Continuous shortwave diathermy with exercise reduces pain and improves function in lateral epicondylitis more than sham diathermy: a randomized controlled trial. *J Bodyw Mov Ther*. 2020;24(1):69-76.

3. Hill J, Lewis M, Mills P, Kielty C. Pulsed short-wave diathermy effects on human fibroblast proliferation. *Arch Phys Med Rehabil*. 2002;83(6):832-836.

4. Ostrowski J, Ely C, Evans H, Bocklund D. Comparison of pulsed shortwave diathermy and continuous short-wave diathermy devices. *Athl Train Sports Health Care*. 2016;8(1):18-26.

5. US Food and Drug Administration. Diathermy. Published 2014. Accessed July 3, 2020. https://www.fda.gov/inspections-compliance-enforcement-and-criminal-investigations/inspection-guides/diathermy

6. Shields N, Gormley J, O'Hare N. Short-wave diathermy: a review of existing clinical trials. *Phys Ther Rev*. 2001;6(2):101-118.

7. Chattanooga. Intelect SWD100 user manual. Published 2009. Accessed July 14, 2020. https://www.djoglobal.com/sites/default/files/Intelect%20SWD100%20Diathermy%20IFU.pdf

8. Watson T. Pulsed shortwave diathermy. Published 2020. Accessed July 14, 2020. http://www.electrotherapy.org/modality/pulsed-shortwave-therapy

Chapter 12

Low-Level Laser Therapy, Infrared Light Therapy, and Ultraviolet Light

KEY TERMS Chromophores | Coherence | Collimation | Cosine law | Erythema | Inverse square law | Light-emitting diode | Minimal erythemal dose | Monochromatic

KEY ABBREVIATIONS FIR | IFR | IR | LED | LLLT | MIRE | UVA | UVB | UVC

CHAPTER OBJECTIVES

1. Describe low-level laser therapy, infrared light, and ultraviolet light as well as their techniques.
2. Explain the physiological effects of low-level laser therapy, infrared, and ultraviolet light.
3. Explain the indications and contraindications for low-level laser therapy, infrared, and ultraviolet light.
4. Demonstrate safety when using each of the listed modalities.
5. Apply knowledge of low-level laser therapy, infrared, and ultraviolet light set-up and parameters to case scenarios.
6. Document low-level laser therapy, infrared, and ultraviolet light interventions correctly in a patient's chart.

INTRODUCTION

Electromagnetic energy is classified by its frequency and its wavelength, which are inversely proportional to each other. Lower-frequency electromagnetic radiation, such as diathermy, ultraviolet (UV), infrared (IFR), visible light, or microwaves are more likely to be used for medical treatments, whereas higher-frequency radiation such as x-rays and gamma rays can break molecular bonds to form ions and inhibit cell division. This chapter will discuss 3 examples of electromagnetic energy modalities; specifically, ones that relate to the use of light to treat tissues.

LOW-LEVEL LASER THERAPY

Many are not aware that LASER is actually an acronym that stands for light amplification of stimulated emissions of radiation. When one thinks of lasers, one may think of science fiction movies or the types of lasers used in surgical procedures, or even laser pointers; the type of laser discussed here is none of these. This section will discuss low-level laser therapy (LLLT), sometimes called a *cold laser*, which is a low-intensity light therapy that yields photochemical effects rather than thermal effects.[1] LLLT applies light at a power range of 10 mW to 500 mW near the IFR area of the light spectrum, and some studies have shown that LLLT can decrease pain and inflammation and promote tissue injury repair.[1] Previous types of lasers used helium-neon or gallium-arsenide as lasing mediums; newer laser models use gallium-aluminum-arsenide as the lasing medium. Wavelengths are measured in nanometers (nm). Helium-neon lasers deliver 632.8 nm, gallium-arsenide lasers deliver 904 nm, and gallium-aluminum-arsenide lasers deliver wavelengths at 780 to 860 nm. While access to lasers in the clinic can be limited, treatment is typically brief and can be easily integrated into a treatment session.

Memolo J.
Therapeutic Agents for the Physical Therapist Assistant
(pp 149-161). © 2022 SLACK Incorporated.

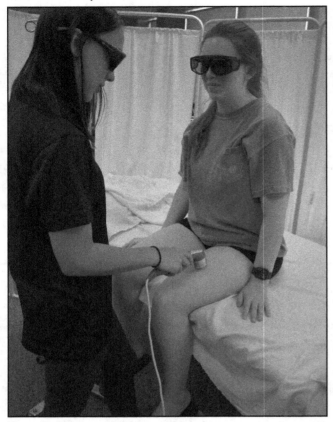

Figure 12-1. Patient and clinician with goggles.

Laser light has 3 qualities that makes it unique: it is monochromatic, coherent, and collimated or directional. *Monochromatic* means that the light is of a single wavelength, which makes it one color. *Coherence* means that the light emitted is of the same wavelength and the waves are in phase with each other, and *collimation* means that the light creates a focused or concentrated beam of light. A benefit of using LLLT is that it can penetrate up to 5 cm.[2]

Physiological Effects of Low-Level Laser Therapy

The brief description of how LLLT affects tissues is that it is absorbed by our cellular photoreceptors, thus causing certain chemical changes.[1] Specifically, it is thought that LLLT acts on the mitochondria, or the power plant of a cell, increasing adenosine triphosphate production. Additionally, when a tissue is injured, nitric oxide produced in our mitochondria displaces oxygen in injured cells. LLLT is thought to reverse this inhibition of oxygenation and cause what some call "light-mediated vasodilation,"[1] meaning LLLT yields all the known physiological effects and benefits of vasodilation. The skin responds well to red and near-IFR light, and photons from LLLT are absorbed by the mitochondrial chromophores in skin cells and activate electron transport, nitric oxide release, blood flow, and

stem cells.[3] LLLT has been shown to promote the proliferation of fibroblasts, endothelial cells, and lymphocytes, all which play a role in tissue repair.[1] Additional physiological effects include angiogenesis and collagen synthesis both in acute and chronic wounds.

With regard to pain control, there are varied opinions on how LLLT decreases pain. LLLT can reach and affect the superficial nerve endings of Aδ and C fibers and thereby affect the pain signal traveling from the superficial nerves to the pain receptors in the brain. LLLT disrupts the transmission of the pain signal and, in this way, the release of substance P is decreased, and the pain signal is delayed.[1] Some studies have likewise shown an increase in endorphin and serotonin levels as a result of LLLT,[4] and some studies show that LLLT can yield both short- and long-term pain reduction. Finally, pain may be reduced because of LLLT's overall reduction of edema and inflammation via the reduction of prostaglandins.[1,5]

Indications and Contraindications of Low-Level Laser Therapy

As mentioned previously, the primary indications for LLLT are pain, inflammation, and tissue injury with the goal of promoting healing. Additional potential indications are improving the tensile strength and reduction of size of scar tissue[3] and possible bone/fracture healing.[6] New research is showing that LLLT may also have positive benefits for patients with traumatic brain injury[7] and spinal cord injury.[8]

While LLLT has many potential benefits, and it is classified as "cold" laser, meaning there is little chance of burning a person with a low-level laser, there are a few contraindications of which to be mindful. The first contraindication is that LLLT should not be administered over the eyes. An additional safety piece is that the patient and the clinician should both wear safety goggles/glasses during an LLLT treatment, and, ideally, the treatment should occur in a separate room or space to prevent potential injury to other patients' eyes. Figure 12-1 demonstrates a patient and clinician wearing protective goggles. Because LLLT has been shown to promote tissue healing and vasodilation, it should not be administered over a site of known cancer in order to avoid metastasis of the cancer. Pregnancy is another contraindication; one should at least not administer LLLT over the abdomen or lower back or during the first trimester.[1] When treating patients with epilepsy, be aware that the light from the laser could trigger a seizure, so at least caution should be exercised in these cases.[1] A seemingly unrelated contraindication includes applying LLLT directly over a tattoo. Some clinicians note that tattoos with red ink are especially susceptible to producing pain or burning when exposed to LLLT. The red ink tends to absorb the light faster and could result in the sensation of pain or burning in that area.[9] Other studies suggest that darker-inked tattoos should, generally, be contraindicated,

Table 12-1

Indications, Contraindications, and Physiological Effects of Low-Level Laser Therapy

Indications	Contraindications	Physiological Effects
Pain reduction	Direct use over eyes; always have goggles	Increases adenosine triphosphate production
Inflammation	Cancer	Reverses deoxygenation in cells; promotes vasodilation
Tissue injury/wound healing	Pregnancy	Promotes nitrous oxide release
Reduce scar size; increase scar tissue tensile strength	Deep vein thrombosis	Activates stem cells
Promote bone healing	Over tattoo with red ink	Promotes proliferation of fibroblasts, endothelial cells, and lymphocytes
	Patients with epilepsy (precaution)	Angiogenesis and collagen synthesis
		Disrupts pain signal traveling on Aδ and C fibers
		Increases endorphin and serotonin levels
		Reduces prostaglandins

and others recommend not performing LLLT over any tattoo.[10] Finally, LLLT should not be used with patients with known deep vein thromboses so as to avoid dislodging a clot and causing a cerebrovascular accident, myocardial infarction, or pulmonary embolism. Table 12-1 lists all of the indications, contraindications, and physiological effects of LLLT.

Application Methods

The application of LLLT depends on a few specific parameters, of which the clinician usually adjusts 2: the energy density (sometimes thought of as the intensity) measured in joules (J) or J/cm^2 and sometimes seen as W/cm^2, and the duration, which is often set by the machine once the energy density is determined. Therefore, most parameter tables will have the diagnosis or treatment goal and then the energy density in J/cm^2. Some units may require one to determine a pulsed vs continuous setting, and if pulsed, specify a pulse rate, but this depends on the machine used. The energy density or intensity varies depending on the treatment goal, but also on the evidence, textbook, or supervising therapist you consult. Some sources indicate that treatment dosages should not exceed 4 J/cm^2 because higher dosages may cause tissue damage.[11] The World Association for Laser Therapy provided a protocol list in 2010 listing parameters for specific diagnoses, and this is sometimes a foundational source to determine treatment protocols.[12] In addition, the Swedish Laser-Medical Society lists parameters for specific diagnoses.[13] What this points to is that more research should be conducted regarding

Table 12-2

Laser Treatment Parameters

Application	Energy Density (J/cm^2)
Pain	Acute: 5 to 50
	Chronic: 4 to 5
Trigger points	Superficial: 1 to 3
	Deep: 1 to 2
Edema reduction	0.1 to 0.5
Inflammation	2 to 4
Tendonopathies	2 to 4
Wound/tissue healing	Superficial: 0.05 to 0.1
	Deep: 0.5 to 2
Scar tissue	4 to 5
Fracture/bone healing	2 to 3

LLLT treatment and parameters, as these can vary widely. Table 12-2 provides some of the recommended treatment parameters for LLLT based on these sources and recent studies. Figure 12-2 provides an example of LLLT parameter set-up. Box 12-1 suggests a research topic regarding LLLT parameters.

In addition to setting the parameters for LLLT, one must also consider how to apply the laser treatment. The laser applicator has light-emitting diode (LED) lights

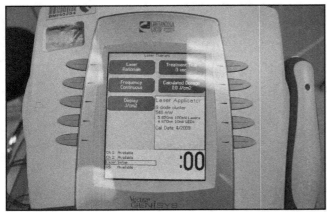

Figure 12-2. LLLT parameter.

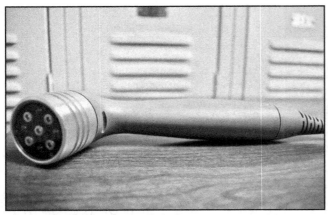

Figure 12-3. Applicator head with diodes.

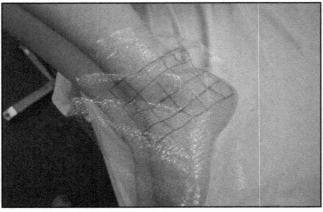

Figure 12-5. Gridding.

(Figure 12-3), and often a button on it that the clinician will press when ready to administer the laser treatment (Figure 12-4). Because a treatment area is usually larger than the size of the laser applicator head, the clinician must administer the laser treatment multiple times. Usually, the treatment area is divided into a grid of squares, with each square being an area that will receive one laser treatment.

Box 12-1
Research Topic

Parameters for the use of LLLT are varied and sometimes contradictory. Conduct your own quick research on the topic; what evidence can you find that supports specific parameters for the treatment of a specific diagnosis? Are there any studies that support parameters for specific diagnoses, such as edema, wound healing, or inflammation?

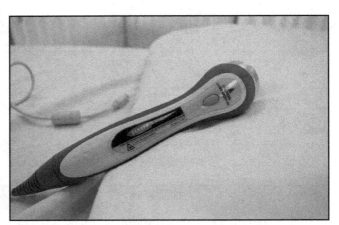

Figure 12-4. Applicator head button.

This technique is called *gridding*, and the clinician will place the applicator head in light contact with the tissue in each square of the grid until the treatment is complete. Bear in mind that the clinician should not actually draw a grid on the patient. If the patient has a wound, one can place a sterile plastic covering over the area to allow for tissue contact. Figure 12-5 shows gridding.

Another technique is called *scanning*, and this is used when contact with the applicator head is inadvisable or difficult. Hold the applicator head at about a 30-degree angle to the tissue and no more than 1 cm from the tissue. Figure 12-6 provides an example of scanning. Wanding is another technique, but it is not recommended because it is difficult to confirm the dosage being administered. In all cases, clean and sanitize the applicator after treatment. Table 12-3 details the steps for administering laser to your patient.

Safety Concerns

As mentioned previously, a significant safety concern is that the patient and the clinician both wear safety glasses during LLLT treatment. This will eliminate the possibility of damaging the eyes during a treatment session. The clinician should adhere to all contraindications, and be mindful if the patient has a tattoo with red or dark ink because this is likely to cause pain or a burning sensation. The good news is that LLLT has few contraindications and generally seems to have only positive effects.

	Table 12-3 Procedures for Applying Low-Level Laser Therapy	
Equipment Needed	<ul><li>Laser unit</li><li>Alcohol wipes</li><li>Towel</li><li>Sheets, pillows</li><li>Treatment table/chair</li></ul>	
Treatment/ Parameters	<ul><li>Confirm patient does not have contraindications to treatment.</li><li>Determine optimal patient position—supine, prone, or seated.</li><li>Remove clothing and jewelry from area.</li><li>Prepare skin area before treatment—clean and wipe dry area.</li><li>Establish correct parameters, typically intensity (energy density) and duration (often set by machine once you set energy density).</li><li>Make sure you and patient are wearing safety goggles.</li><li>Begin treatment; apply laser by pressing button on applicator head every time administering laser using a gridding or scanning technique.</li><li>Check patient's skin and ask for feedback after treatment.</li></ul>	
Safety Considerations	<ul><li>Monitor patient's response (verbally and visually) during treatment session.</li><li>Make sure you and patient are wearing goggles and ideally are in an isolated location.</li></ul>	
Advantages	<ul><li>Patient usually does not feel anything during treatment</li><li>Treatment session is brief and easily worked in to a therapy appointment</li></ul>	
Disadvantages	<ul><li>Parameters can vary depending on unit and type of laser</li><li>Some insurance companies may not reimburse for laser; time component may not allow for billing</li></ul>	

INFRARED LIGHT

IFR light or infrared radiation (IR) is another electromagnetic energy modality that can produce thermal effects. Sometimes IFR is further subclassified as far (FIR) or near (NIR) infrared light. FIR is correlated with longer wavelengths; NIR has shorter wavelengths. Both types are used therapeutically to yield certain benefits to the tissues and can be administered with lamps, LEDs, or IFR saunas. There are even pieces of clothing with FIR-emitting nanoparticles to cause its health benefits.[14] It is thought that IFR light can possibly penetrate deeper than other thermal modalities, up to 1.5 inches (3.8 cm) in the case of FIR.[15]

Physiological Effects of Infrared Light

Electromagnetic energy is thought to alter cell membrane potentials and alter mitochondrial metabolism.[14] In the case of FIR, the energy is absorbed and causes vibration in the cellular water molecules. This vibration can cause what is normally felt as a gentle heat in the tissues, and these effects can be longer lasting than those of other thermal modalities.[14] As with other thermal modalities, the effects of IFR

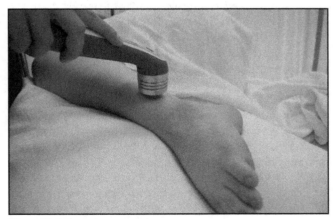

Figure 12-6. Scanning.

can be vasodilation, increased blood flow, pain reduction via the Gate Control theory, as well as improved healing.

There are other, nonthermal effects of IFR light that are less understood. We learned previously that LLLT causes vasodilation and increased blood flow, but not because of the generation of heat. Instead, the mitochondrial chromophores absorb the red light and cause the loss of nitrous

Box 12-2
Research Topic

Conduct some research on the topic of monochromatic infrared radiation energy (MIRE; brand name Anodyne) and its effects on peripheral neuropathy. How recent is the research? What do the studies conclude regarding its use? What level(s) of evidence are the studies you can find?

oxide, which then allows for increased electron transport, oxygen consumption, and adenosine triphosphate production.[14] It is thought, then, that IFR light works in a similar way. Some studies have shown that FIR increases blood flow and promotes wound healing in rats by increasing collagen content and myofibroblast production.[14]

Indications and Contraindications of Infrared Light

Some recent studies have shown that FIR and NIR can be used to promote wound healing, decrease pain, increase circulation, decrease joint stiffness, and, in the case of FIR, to possibly stimulate mesenchymal and cardiac stem cells in patients with chronic heart disease.[16] In addition, IFR light has been used to improve the pain, numbness, and tingling sensations in patients with neuropathy via monochromatic IFR light, but the research is less clear regarding whether IFR is actually effective.[17] Box 12-2 provides a research opportunity on this topic. FIR has also been trialed to reduce the pain and inflammation of rheumatoid arthritis, and to even improve quality of sleep.[14] As in the case of LLLT, one has to be careful to avoid the idea that IFR has a cure-all capability and continue studies to determine its true effects and benefits.

Contraindications for IFR light are few, but they include the application of IFR for any acute injury. One should take steps to reduce the risk of burning the patient. In the case of IFR lights, it is important to keep the light a sufficient distance away from the tissue being treated. The rationale for this is the inverse square law, which states that the farther away an object is from a light source, the less radiation or light it will receive. Figures 12-7 and 12-8 show the difference of the lamp being farther and closer to the tissue. Additionally, the clinician should cover any other tissue they do not want to expose to the IFR light with dry towels, and some texts suggest covering the treatment area with a moist towel to reduce the risk of burns. An additional contraindication includes patients with deep vein thromboses because increased circulation can cause an increased risk of the thrombus becoming an embolus. Table 12-4 lists the indications and contraindications for IFR light.

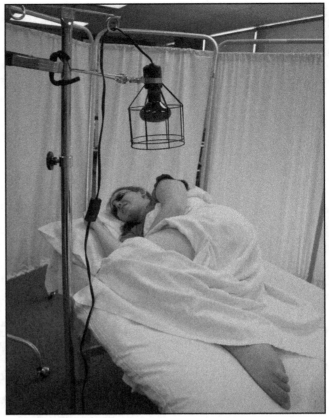

Figure 12-7. Light closer to patient.

Application Methods

In the case of IFR light therapy via LEDs, which goes by the brand name of Anodyne Therapy but is also referred to as *monochromatic infrared radiation energy* (MIRE), it is usually administered for 30 to 45 minutes on the specified treatment area.[18] If using a traditional IFR lamp, treatment time may be up to 15 to 30 minutes, with care to check the skin 5 minutes after beginning the treatment and heeding the patient's complaints of the lamp feeling too hot. Previously mentioned precautions of draping any nontreatment areas with dry towels are advised (Figure 12-9). Ideally, the lamp should be at a 90-degree angle, or perpendicular, to the tissue. This is because the cosine law states that the smaller the angle between the light ray and a right angle, the less light and radiation will be reflected and the more will be absorbed. Figure 12-10 shows the difference when the light is at a 45-degree angle. Depending on the lamp, the light could be up to 20 inches (51 cm) away from the tissue to decrease the risk of burning. Table 12-5 offers the procedure for applying IFR light to a patient.

Table 12-4
Indications, Contraindications, and Physiological Effects of Infrared Light

Indications	Contraindications	Physiological Effects
Wound healing	Acute injury	Alters mitochondrial metabolism
Pain	Potential for burns	Causes molecular vibration and heat
Decreased circulation	Deep vein thrombosis	Vasodilation
Joint stiffness		Increased blood flow
Neuropathy		Pain reduction via Gate Control theory
Rheumatoid arthritis		Increases collagen and myofibroblast production
Sleep deficits		Mitochondrial chromophores absorb the red light and cause the loss of nitric oxide, promoting electron transport, oxygen consumption, and adenosine triphosphate production
		Stimulate stem cells

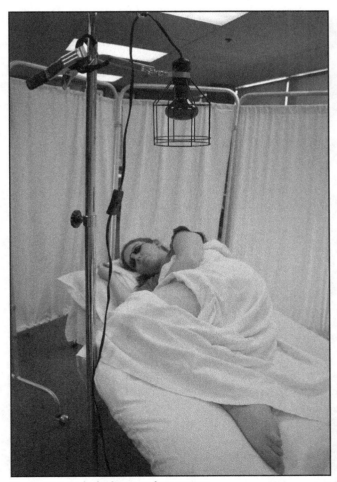

Figure 12-8. Light farther away from patient.

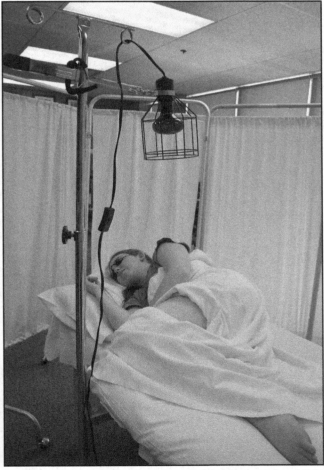

Figure 12-9. Patient with only the treatment area exposed and light set-up.

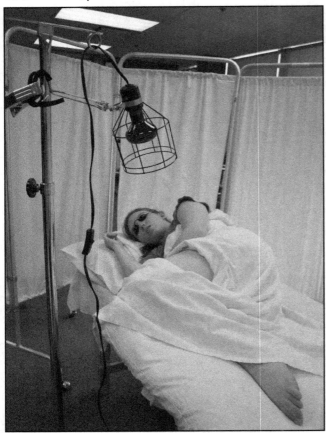

Figure 12-10. Patient with the light at a 45-degree angle.

Safety Concerns

Patients may need to wear protective glasses, as prolonged exposure of the eyes to IFR light can cause eye damage. Excessive exposure can also cause photoaging (skin aging as a result of light exposure), and most significantly, IFR light does run the risk of burning the patient's skin, so care must be taken during its use.

ULTRAVIOLET LIGHT

One may think about getting a suntan or a sunburn when thinking about UV light, or the importance of wearing sunscreen to prevent skin cancer. UV light is divided into 3 categories: UVA, UVB, and UVC. All 3 types are emitted by the sun, but only UVA and UVB light reaches Earth. UVA and UVB light can both be dangerous to the tissue if exposure is prolonged; UVA can cause skin aging and UVB light is associated both with the production of vitamin D and skin cancer. UVC light has a shorter wavelength but can still damage tissues with excessive exposure. However, it has also been shown to be effective in the treatment of wounds, particularly those with infection. UVC is

also used to treat certain skin conditions, such as psoriasis or acne, but this is not within the physical therapist assistant's scope of practice.

Physiological Effects of Ultraviolet Light

While UVA and UVB light have known dangerous effects on tissues (think skin aging, sunburns, and skin cancer), UVC light has been shown to promote wound healing in a variety of ways. Primarily, UVC is germicidal, meaning it is an effective way to treat infected wounds, including those colonized by methicillin-resistant *Staphylococcus aureus*.[19] UVC light damages the genetic material in the nucleus of a cell; its shorter wavelength allows it to be absorbed by the nucleic acids of a micro-organism and is, therefore, lethal.[20] As a result, the DNA and RNA are damaged, and the micro-organism either cannot replicate or its replication is defected, making it less viable.[20]

UVC light has also been studied for its potential effects on promoting wound reepithelialization. Use of UVC light in the treatment of wounds has shown some effects of promoting granulation tissue formation as well as the sloughing of necrotic tissue.[20] It is also hypothesized that the use of UVC light in the treatment of wounds can protect the new tissue from UV exposure by encouraging the production of melanin.[20]

Indications and Contraindications of Ultraviolet Light

As mentioned, UVC is primarily used in physical therapy as a means to treat wounds. Wounds that are already infected or at a high risk for infection are indicated for the use of UVC, but chronic or nonhealing wounds may also benefit from UVC light use.

Contraindications are few, but it is important to check with your patient to avoid potential injury. Because UVC light has the potential of carcinogenic effects, some clinicians are hesitant to use UVC light; however, no studies have yet shown UVC light use in the treatment of wounds to cause skin cancer. One would want to limit the treatment times to avoid this possible side effect. Because UVC is a light source, patient and clinician should both wear protective eyewear to avoid damage to the retinas. Clinicians should consider patients who are photosensitive, such as patients with systemic lupus erythematosus, or those taking medications that make them photosensitive, such as tetracycline, at least a precaution for the use of UVC light. Likewise, patients who either currently have skin cancer, have a history of skin cancer, or are at a high risk for skin cancer, should exercise caution with UVC use. Table 12-6 lists the indications, contraindications, and physiological effects of UV light.

	Table 12-5 Procedures for Applying Infrared Light
Equipment Needed	• Infrared lamp, Anodyne unit, etc • Protective goggles • Alcohol wipes • Towel • Sheets, pillows • Treatment table/chair
Treatment/ Parameters	• Confirm patient does not have contraindications to treatment. • Determine optimal patient position—supine, prone, or seated. • Remove clothing and jewelry from area. • Prepare skin area before treatment—clean and wipe dry area. • Establish correct parameters, including distance of lamp (~ 20 inches [51 cm]), and angle of lamp to tissues (ideally perpendicular). • Make sure you and patient are wearing safety goggles. • Drape nontreatment areas with dry towels. • Begin treatment; provide patient a call light/bell. Check on patient 5 min after treatment begins. • Patient can receive treatment for 15 to 30 min. • Check patient's skin and ask for feedback after treatment.
Safety Considerations	• Monitor patient's response (verbally and visually) during treatment session. • Make sure you and patient are wearing goggles and other tissue is protected by dry towels. • May need to move lamp farther away if patient becomes too warm.
Advantages	• Patient usually feels gentle warmth • No contact required during treatment • Good to treat contoured areas • Patient and therapist can monitor skin during treatment
Disadvantages	• Parameters can vary depending on unit and type of laser • Difficult to ensure consistent and equal heating to specific area • Some insurance companies may not reimburse for laser; time component may not allow for billing

Application Methods

When administering UV light to a patient, one may need to determine the correct dosage. To do that, first establish the patient's minimal erythemal dose (MED), which is the amount of UV light exposure that will result in minimal erythema (redness) to the patient's skin within a few hours of exposure. To do this, the clinician exposes several areas of the patient's skin using a piece of paper or cardboard with 5 holes cut out, usually on the underside of the forearm, to progressively longer durations of UV light. An example of this is shown in Figure 12-11. The light should be held at a 90-degree angle to the tissue being tested. Each section will be labeled, and the therapist will record the time for each exposure. The holes should be exposed in 15-second increments of 15, 30, 45, 60, and 75 seconds (meaning the first exposed hole will receive a total of 75 seconds of exposure and the last exposed hole will receive 15 seconds of exposure). All other body parts will be draped to protect the tissue.[21] In this way, the first hole will have the longest exposure and the last hole will have the shortest. In 24 to 48 hours, the therapist checks the skin. Skin that shows redness for the least amount of time without being burned is determined to be the MED. Then what? The clinician now knows the duration of UV light the patient can be exposed to without burning, so all future UV treatments should be shorter than that time.

Table 12-6

Indications, Contraindications, and Physiological Effects of Ultraviolet Light

Indications	Contraindications	Physiological Effects
Wounds	Photosensitive patients or those taking medications that would make them photosensitive	Damages DNA and RNA in nucleus or nucleic acids of microorganisms' cells, making them unable to replicate or unviable
Certain skin conditions (acne, psoriasis)—not physical therapist/physical therapist assistant scope of practice	Patients with systemic lupus erythematosus	Promotes wound epithelialization, granulation tissue to form, and sloughing of necrotic tissue
	Patients with current skin cancer or at higher risk for skin cancer (patients should be checked regularly)	Protects new tissue with production of melanin
	Prolonged use could have carcinogenic effects	Increased pigmentation
	Protect eyes when using UVC; can cause retinal damage	Vitamin D production
	Patients with tuberculosis	

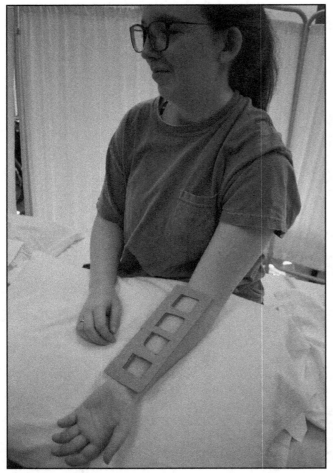

Figure 12-11. MED set-up.

In some cases, however, an MED is not required. Most studies indicate that a treatment time of 90 to 180 seconds is sufficient to kill bacteria.[19,22] If one is using a portable UVC light, one with a specific energy output (often measured in mW/cm^2) or a specific dose (often measured in mJ/cm^2), the treatment requires the application of UVC light from the lamp 1 inch (2.5 cm) away from the wound, perpendicular to the wound base.[22] Some clinicians recommend applying petroleum jelly to the periwound area; however, other studies suggest that periwound exposure can allow for epithelial cell growth to help the wound close.[22] One would still aim to cover the rest of the tissue to protect it, and clinician and patient should both wear protective glasses. See Table 12-7 for details on applying UV light.

Safety Concerns

The primary safety concerns of UVC light relate to protecting the eyes, protecting the tissue not being treated, and monitoring the tissue response. If one is able, it is helpful to establish the MED to prevent tissue injury.

DOCUMENTATION

The use of electromagnetic light modalities requires the inclusion of certain parameters. As with other modalities, be sure to include the patient positioning and the body part being treated. Then include the parameters specific to that modality. In the case of LLLT, include the intensity in J/cm^2; if using IFR, include the power of the lamp, distance of the lamp from the tissue, and angle of the lamp to the tissue. In the case of UVC light, include the output or

	Table 12-7
	Procedures for Applying Ultraviolet C Light
Equipment Needed	• UVC light • Alcohol wipes • Towel • Sheets, pillows • Treatment table/chair
Treatment/ Parameters	• Confirm patient does not have contraindications to treatment. • Determine optimal patient position—supine, prone, or seated. • Remove clothing and jewelry from area. • Prepare skin area before treatment—clean and wipe dry area. • Establish correct parameters, typically intensity (energy density) and duration (often set by machine once you set energy density). You may also need to establish MED to determine parameters. • To establish MED: Use cardboard or paper with 5 holes cut out. Label each hole 1 to 5. Use towels to expose on first hole, and expose × 15 sec with lamp at 90-degree angle. Then expose second hole (with first still exposed) × 15 sec; continue until all holes exposed. Check back 24 hours later to determine MED, or smallest dose that yielded erythema in 8 hours but fades within 24 hours. • Make sure you and patient are wearing safety goggles. • Check patient's skin and ask for feedback after treatment.
Safety Considerations	• Monitor patient's response (verbally and visually) during treatment session. • Make sure you and patient are wearing goggles and ideally are in an isolated location.
Advantages	• Patient usually does not feel anything during treatment • UVC light is cheaper and safer than using antibiotics
Disadvantages	• Parameters can vary depending on unit • Some insurance companies may not reimburse for UVC light • Research is spotty on its use or effectiveness • May not be able to reach infections in deeper tissues

intensity of the lamp, if known, and the distance and angle of the lamp. In all cases, include the duration of the treatment in seconds or minutes. See the following examples of documentation for these modalities.

Diagnosis: Patient has left knee bursitis with pain at a 6/10 during ambulation and stair negotiation.

O: Patient received LLLT at 780 to 860 nm with 4 J/cm^2 × 2 minutes using a gridding technique to the left anterior knee.

Diagnosis: Patient has a stage IV sacral pressure injury with noted necrosis and yellow slough at 3 o'clock and 5 o'clock areas, respectively. Wound measures at 2.7 cm × 2.1 cm × 1.2 cm.

O: Patient received UVC light × 180 seconds to sacral wound base with lamp held at 90-degree angle and 1 inch (2.5 cm) away from wound. All other areas draped.

CONCLUSION

Electromagnetic energy modalities such as LLLT, IFR, and UV light each offers its own potential benefits to patient care. LLLT has been shown to have several positive effects such as reducing pain and promoting healing, but more research needs to be conducted to determine the most effective parameters and to better understand the mechanisms of how it works. Similarly, IFR and UV light have potentially positive effects on the body's tissues, including pain reduction and wound healing, but more research is needed to support these claims and to determine parameters.

Review Questions

1. What are the indications and contraindications of laser?
2. Discuss the physiological effects of laser.
3. Compare gridding and scanning as the main techniques of application of laser.
4. Describe at least 2 ways IFR light affects the body physiologically.
5. What are the main safety considerations when applying IFR light?
6. What is the primary physical therapy indication for UVC light?
7. Describe the process of establishing an MED.
8. Discuss the contraindications for UVC light treatment.
9. You have a patient who has a stage III pressure injury on her sacrum. The wound measures 2.1 mm × 1.3 mm × 0.9 mm, and she has some minimal pain in the peri-wound area. What light-based modality do you think would be best for this patient? Why? What parameters or treatment protocol would you recommend?
10. Your patient has right lateral epicondylitis of the elbow with 7/10 pain when lifting with that arm or gripping. If you were to apply LLLT to this area, what treatment parameters and set-up would you recommend? How would you document this treatment?

Case Study 1

Your patient is an 85-year-old woman with a nonhealing, infected stage IV wound on her sacrum. She is already receiving ultrasound to the area, but the ensuing infection has slowed her progress. Your supervising physical therapist wants you to use UVC light to assist in the healing process.
1. What tissues are injured/affected?
2. What safety precautions must you follow when administering UV light?
3. What are the contraindications for UV light?
4. What other therapeutic interventions would you recommend for this patient? Why?

Case Study 2

You are working with a 68-year-old man with rheumatoid arthritis in his hands and wrists. He is a painter and finds it difficult to hold his paintbrushes now. He takes ibuprofen but does not want to take more than he already takes. The goal is to reduce the pain and inflammation so he can resume his painting.

1. What tissues are affected?
2. What parameter(s) of LLLT would you select for this patient? What treatment method would you use?
3. What other therapeutic intervention(s) would you recommend for this patient? Why?
4. What are the contraindications for LLLT?

References

1. Cotler HB, Chow RT, Hamblin MR, Carroll J. The use of low level laser therapy (LLLT) for musculoskeletal pain. *MOJ Orthop Rheumatol.* 2015;2(5):00068.
2. DJO Global. Low level laser therapy 101. Accessed July 17, 2020. https://www.djoglobal.com/sites/default/files/Low%20Level%20Laser%20Therapy%20101.pdf
3. Avci P, Gupta A, Sadasivam M, et al. Low-level laser (light) therapy (LLLT) in skin: stimulating, healing, restoring. *Semin Cutan Med Surg.* 2013;32(1):41-52.
4. Lamba D. To evaluate the efficacy of 780 nm low level laser therapy for the treatment of plantar fasciitis in South Western Ethiopia. *Indian J Physiother Occup Ther.* 2019;13(2):231-235.
5. Moreira SH, Pazzini JM, Álvarez JLG, et al. Evaluation of angiogenesis, inflammation, and healing on irradiated skin graft with low-level laser therapy in rats. *Lasers Med Sci.* 2020;35(5):1103-1109.
6. Ip D. Enhanced healing and bone re-modelling by low-level laser therapy for rapid pain control in pediatric fractures. *Int J Pain Management.* 2019;1(1):23-28.
7. da Cruz Ribeiro Poiani G, Zaninotto AL, Costa Carneiro AM, et al. Photobiomodulation using low-level laser therapy (LLLT) for patients with chronic traumatic brain injury: a randomized controlled trial study protocol. *Trials.* 2018;19:17.
8. de Silva FC, Gomes AO, da Costa Palacio PR, et al. Photobiomodulation improves motor response in patients with spinal cord injury submitted to electromyographic evaluation: randomized clinical trial. *Lasers Med Sci.* 2018;33(4):883-890.
9. Thor. What are the PBM therapy contra-indications? Published 2020. Accessed July 17, 2020. https://www.thorlaser.com/LLLT/contraindications.htm
10. Ingenito T. Low level light therapy and tattoos: a case report. *J Bodyw Mov Ther.* 2016;20(4):748-750.
11. Laakso L, Richardson C, Cramond T. Factors affecting low level laser therapy. *Aust J Physiother.* 1993;39(2):95-99.
12. World Association for Laser Therapy. Dosage recommendations. Published 2010. Accessed July 22, 2020. https://waltza.co.za/documentation-links/recommendations/dosage-recommendations/
13. Energy Laser. Guidelines for treatment with laser therapy. Published 2019. Accessed July 22, 2020. https://energy-laser.com/guide-lines-for-treatment-with-laser-therapy/
14. Vatansever F, Hamblin MR. Far infrared radiation (FIR): its biological effects and medical applications. *Photonics Lasers Med.* 2012;4:255-266.

15. Ervolino F, Gazze R. Far infrared wavelength treatment for low back pain: evaluation of a non-invasive device. *Work.* 2016;53(1):157-162.

16. Tsai SR, Hamblin MR. Biological effects and medical applications of infrared radiation. *J Photochem Photobiol B.* 2017;170:197-207.

17. Cabral Robinson C, Da Silva Klahr P, Stein C, Falavigna M, Sbruzzi G, Della Méa Plentz R. Effects of monochromatic infrared phototherapy in patients with diabetic peripheral neuropathy: a systematic review and meta-analysis of randomized controlled trials. *Braz J Phys Ther.* 2017;21(4):233-243.

18. Moda. Anodyne Therapy (Monochromatic Infrared Energy). Published 2019. Accessed July 24, 2020. https://www.moda-health.com/pdfs/med_criteria/Anodyne.pdf

19. Thai TP, Keast DH, Campbell KE, Woodbury MG, Houghton PE. Effect of ultraviolet light C on bacterial colonization in chronic wounds. *Ostomy Wound Manage.* 2005;51(10):32-38.

20. Dai T, Vrahas MS, Murray CK, Hamblin MR. Ultraviolet C irradiation: an alternative antimicrobial approach to localized infections? *Expert Rev Anti Infect Ther.* 2012;10(2):185-195.

21. Heckman C, Chandler R, Kloss J, et al. Minimal erythema dose (MED) testing. *J Vis Exp.* 2013;(75):e50175.

22. Yarboro D, Millar A, Smith R. The effects of ultraviolet C irradiation in the treatment of chronic wounds: a retrospective, descriptive study. *Wound Manag Prev.* 2019;65(7):16-22.

Glossary

A

Absolute refractory period: the period of time immediately after nerve depolarization when no action potential can be generated.

Accommodation: temporary increase in the threshold to nerve excitation.

Acoustic streaming: steady, circular flow of cellular fluids induced by ultrasound.

Action potential (AP): the rapid depolarization and repolarization of a nerve that occurs in response to a stimulus and transmits along an axon.

Acute pain: pain that has a sudden onset and less than 6 months' duration; usually has an easily identifiable cause.

Alternating current (AC): see *biphasic current.*

Ampere (A, amp): a unit of electric current equal to a flow of one coulomb per second.

Amplitude: the maximum value of current or voltage; interchangeable with *intensity.*

Analgesia: insensibility to pain, such as when one takes painkillers.

Anesthesia: controlled, temporary loss of sensation or awareness for the use of pain relief (as when using cryotherapy).

Anode: the positive electrode.

Anulus fibrosus: ring of fibrocartilage that forms the outer layer of the intervertebral disc.

Attenuation: Decrease in ultrasound intensity as ultrasound travels through tissue.

B

Beam nonuniformity rate (BNR): the ratio of the spatial peak intensity to the spatial average intensity; usually 5:1 or 6:1.

Biphasic current (also alternating current): uninterrupted, bidirectional flow of ions; can be burst modulated as in Russian current or amplitude modulated as in interferential current.

Buoyancy: the upward force on an object immersed in fluid that is equal to the weight of the fluid it displaces, making it float or appear lighter.

163

Memolo J.
Therapeutic Agents for the Physical Therapist Assistant
(pp 163-168). © 2022 SLACK Incorporated.

C

Capacitance (diathermy): uses 2 plates that create an electromagnetic field in which the patient is a part of the electrical current.

Cathode: the negative electrode.

Cavitation: the formation, growth, and pulsation of gas-filled bubbles caused by ultrasound, made smaller during compression and larger during rarefaction. May be stable, during which the bubbles oscillate but do not burst (as seen in nonthermal ultrasound), or unstable, in which the bubbles implode and can cause temperature increase and the formation of free radicals.

Chromophores: light-absorbing parts of a molecule that give it color.

Chronic pain: pain that persists beyond the usual amount of time for tissue healing to occur (> 6 months).

Clonus: multiple rhythmic oscillations or beats in the resistance of a muscle responding to a quick stretch.

Coherence: when the waves that make up a light are in phase with each other, such as with lasers.

Collimation: when light has parallel waves.

Conduction: heat transfer as a result of energy exchange by direct collision between molecules of 2 materials at different temperatures. Heat is transferred by conduction when the materials are in contact with each other.

Conductors: an object or type of material that allows for the flow of electrical current in one or more directions, such as metal.

Continuous (diathermy): when the diathermy machine is on 100% of the time and the unit is generating either the alternating electric field or magnetic current all of the time.

Continuous (ultrasound): continuous delivery of ultrasound during the treatment period (no off time).

Convection: heat transfer through direct contact of a circulating medium with a material of a different temperature.

Conversion: heat transfer by the conversion of a nonthermal form of energy, such as electrical, mechanical, or chemical energy, into heat.

Cosine law: states that the smaller the angle between the ray and a right angle, the less radiation will be reflected and the greater will be absorbed.

Cryotherapy: the therapeutic use of cold.

(electrical) Current: the flow of electric charge past a point or region; the flow of charged particles.

D

Debridement: removal of foreign material or dead, damaged, or infected tissue from a wound to promote healing.

Deep somatic pain: occurs when stimuli activate deep pain receptors, such as in the tendons, joints, bones, and deeper muscles; usually feels like aching.

Deep vein thrombosis (DVT): blood clot in a deep vein.

Depolarization: the reversing of the resting potential in excitable cell membranes, where the inside of the cell becomes more positive compared to the outside.

Direct current (DC): continuous, unidirectional flow of charged particles; commonly used for iontophoresis and wound care.

Duty cycle: the proportion of the total treatment time that ultrasound is on. Expressed as a percentage (20%, 100%) or a ratio (20% = 1:5 duty cycle).

E

Edema: swelling that results from the accumulation of fluids in interstitial spaces.

Effective radiation area (ERA): area of the transducer from which the ultrasound energy radiates, as a result of the crystal not vibrating uniformly. Always smaller than the transducer head.

Effleurage: massage technique in which the clinician's hands glide over the skin without affecting the deeper muscle tissues.

Electrical stimulation: use of electrical current to induce motor or sensory effects on the tissue.

Electromagnetic agents: physical agents that apply energy to the patient in the form of electromagnetic radiation or electrical current.

Endorphins: endogenous, opiate-like peptides that reduce the perception of pain by binding to the opiate receptors in the nervous system.

Erythema: redness of the skin.

Eschar: dead tissue or a scab that forms on a wound; usually needs to be debrided to promote wound healing.

Evidence-based research: using current research/evidence from high-level sources to support clinical interventions.

Exudate: fluid that emerges from a wound that has high protein content and white blood cells or solid materials from the wound.

F

Facet joints: small, cartilage-lined points of contact where each vertebra meets the one above and below it; allow the spine to flex during movement.

Fascia: connective tissue that surrounds muscles, tendons, nerves, bones, and organs, composed primarily of collagen.

Flaccidity: lack of tone or absence of resistance to a passive stretch within the middle range of the muscle's length.

Foramina: holes in bone, such as in the spine.

Frequency: in ultrasound, the number of compression/rarefaction cycles per unit of time, expressed in cycles/second, or hertz (Hz). Usually either 1 MHz or 3 MHz. The higher the frequency, the more superficial penetration. In electromagnetic energy, it is the number of waves per unit of time, measured in Hz, or waves/second.

Friction massage: massage technique used to mechanically loosen adhesions of underlying tissue or scar tissue.

G

Gate Control theory: theory by Melzack and Wall[1] that pain is modulated at the spinal cord level by the use of nonnoxious afferent sensory input to "gate" the pain.

Granulation tissue: tissue with new blood vessels, connective tissue, fibroblasts, and inflammatory cells that fill a wound when it first begins to heal; usually deep pink or red (hamburger meat) in appearance.

H

Hunting response: a process of alternating vasoconstriction and vasodilation during exposure to cold, especially to the extremities; initial cold exposure yields vasoconstriction, but several minutes after exposure, blood vessels begin to vasodilate. This is followed by a repetition of this process.

Hydrostatic pressure: the pressure exerted by a fluid on the body immersed in that fluid; increases with increased depth and the amount of immersion.

Hydrotherapy: the therapeutic use of water.

Hypertonic: has excessive tone in the muscle or resistant to stretch.

Hypotonic: has less than normal tone in the muscle or not resistant to stretch.

I

Impedance: the total frequency-dependent opposition to current flow, noted as Z and measured in ohms.

Inductance (diathermy): diathermy that uses a drum or metal coil to create an alternating electromagnetic field to create friction and heat. The patient is not a part of the electrical current.

Insulators: a material in which an electrical current does not or cannot flow freely.

Intermittent (compression): pressure that is alternately applied and released, usually using a pneumatic pump.

Intermittent (traction): traction in which the force of the pull varies every few seconds.

Intervertebral disc: a layer of cartilage separating adjacent vertebrae in the spine that serves as a shock absorber and allows for slight mobility in the spine.

Inverse square law: law that states that the intensity of heat at the skin surface will be greater at a closer distance than at a farther distance; the intensity of radiation striking a surface varies inversely with the square of the distance from the source.

L

Levels of evidence: a ranking system used to describe the strength of the results of clinical trials or research studies.

Light-emitting diode (LED): semiconductor diode light source that produces relatively low-power light in a range of frequencies; may appear to be one color but will have a range of wavelengths and will not be coherent or collimated.

Long-stretch bandage: an elastic bandage that can extend by 100% to 200% and provides a high resting pressure.

Lymphatic fluid: rich in protein, water, and macrophages, this fluid is removed from interstitial spaces via the lymphatic system and returned to the venous system.

Lymphedema: swelling caused by the excess of lymphatic fluid in interstitial spaces.

M

Maceration: when tissue absorbs or is immersed in water for a prolonged period of time and becomes softer and more prone to injury or of a wound expanding, such as being in a bath too long or wearing a brief that is not changed often enough.

Manual traction: the use of force by the therapist to distract joints.

Mechanical agents: physical agents that apply force to increase or decrease pressure on the body.

Mechanical effects (massage): massage techniques that stretch or elongate or mobilize adhesions.

Microstreaming: microscale eddying that takes place during any small, vibrating object; occurs around gas bubbles that oscillate during cavitation.

Minimal erythemal dose (MED): the smallest dose of ultraviolet light that produces redness in the skin that appears within 8 hours but disappears within 24 hours of exposure.

Monochromatic: light of a single frequency, wavelength, and color, such as laser light.

Monophasic current: can also refer to direct current, but is interrupted and not continuous (eg, pulsed).

Myofascial release: a group of techniques that relieves soft tissue from the grip of tight fascia.

N

Nociceptors: nerves that are activated by noxious stimuli, causing the sensation of pain.

Nosocomial: an infection acquired while in a hospital or facility for a different reason (such as acquiring pneumonia while in the hospital for a knee replacement surgery).

Nucleus pulposus: the elastic, pulpy substance found at the center of an intervertebral disc.

O

Ohm: unit of an electrical current that is the electrical resistance between 2 points of a conductor.

Osmotic pressure: pressure determined by the concentration of proteins in and out of blood vessels that contributes to the movement of fluid in or out of the blood or lymph vessels.

Overload principle: strengthening principle that states the greater the load placed on the muscle and the higher the force of contraction, the stronger the muscle will become.

P

Petrissage: kneading manipulations during massage when one presses and rolls the muscles or tissue under the fingers.

Phase duration: duration of one phase of a pulse; usually expressed in microseconds (μs) or milliseconds (ms).

PICO(T): establishing a research question that reflects each of the following: patient/problem, intervention, comparison, outcome, and time.

Piezoelectric: able to generate electricity in response to a mechanical force or being able to change shape in response to an electrical current, such as in ultrasound.

Plan of care: written plan created by the supervising physical therapist related to the specific goals and services provided to the patient for optimal health and outcomes.

Positional traction: prolonged specific positioning of the body to place tension or create a distractive force on the lumbar spine.

Propagation: an action potential moves as a wave along an axon and spreads out, depolarizing adjacent sections of its membrane.

Pulsatile current: flow of charged particles stops periodically for short time; pulses can occur individually or in series.

Pulse duration: the time from the beginning of a first phase of a pulse to the end of the last phase of a pulse; expressed in microseconds (μs).

Pulsed (diathermy): when the diathermy machine has an on and off time, where the output is on at consistent intervals or pulses, where the off time is longer than the on time.

Pulsed (ultrasound): intermittent delivery of ultrasound during the treatment time. Minimizes the thermal effects.

Purulent: pus in a wound; opaque wound fluid that has white blood cells, tissue debris, and micro-organisms. Typically indicates infection.

Q

Qualitative (studies): research/studies that use and look at nonstatistical data such as interviews or questionnaires to support a thesis.

Quantitative (studies): research/studies that use and look at statistical, mathematical data to support a thesis.

R

Radiating pain: pain that begins in one area of the body and spreads to other areas, often following along a specific nerve (such as in sciatica).

Radiation: transfer of energy from one material to another without the need of direct contact or an intervening medium.

Referred pain: pain that is experienced in one area when the damage or injury has occurred in a different area of the body.

Reflection: the redirection of a beam away from a surface at an angle equal and opposite to the angle of incidence; there is 100% reflection when ultrasound meets air and none with coupling medium use.

Reflexive effects (massage): massage techniques that modulate pain, increase circulation, and increase metabolism.

Refraction: the redirection of a wave at an interface; the ultrasound wave enters the tissue at one angle and continues through the tissue at another angle.

Repolarization: the return of a cell membrane potential to its resting membrane potential after depolarization.

Resistance (electrical current): a material's opposition to the flow of electrical current; noted as R and measured in ohms.

Resistance (hydrotherapy): a force counter to the direction of movement; proportional to the relative speed of the body in water and the water's motion and to the frontal areas of the body in contact with the water.

Resting membrane potential: when a neuron is at rest, and the electrical difference between the inside and the outside of a neuron, with the inside being more negative compared to the outside.

Resting pressure: pressure exerted by an elastic bandage when put on stretch.

Rigidity: abnormal, hypertonic state when muscles are stiff or immovable and are resistant to stretch regardless of velocity or direction.

S

Sclerotome: a specific section of bone innervated by a nerve root; results in deep bone pain if injured.

Self-traction: uses gravity and the weight of the patient's body to exert a distractive force.

Short-stretch bandage: a bandage with low elasticity that provides a low resting pressure but a high working pressure during muscle activity.

Spasticity: muscle hypertonicity and increased tendon reflexes in which quicker passive stretches elicit greater resistance than slower stretches.

Spatial average temporal average intensity (SATA): the spatial average intensity of the ultrasound averaged over the on and off time of the pulse.

Spatial average temporal peak intensity (SATP): the spatial average intensity of the ultrasound during the on time of the pulse, the measure of the amount of energy delivered to the tissue.

Specificity (principle): strength gains are specific to the type of training conducted.

Spinal nerve roots: where both dorsal (afferent) and ventral (efferent) nerves emerge from the spinal cord.

Static (compression): steady application of compression to a tissue.

Static (traction): traction in which the same force is applied throughout the treatment session.

Sweep: frequency modulation of an interferential current.

T

Tapotement: also called *percussion*; brisk blows with relaxed hands in alternating movements to stimulate subcutaneous structures during massage.

Therapeutic agents: the administration of thermal, sound, mechanical, electrical, electromagnetic, or light energies for therapeutic effects, such as to decrease pain, increase range of motion, or improve tissue healing.

Thermal agents: physical agents that cause an increase or decrease in tissue temperature.

Thermal conductivity: the rate at which a material transfers heat via conduction.

Thermotherapy: the therapeutic application of heat.

Trigger points: focal, hyperirritable points along skeletal muscle that produce local and referred pain, often associated with musculoskeletal disorders.

V

Vasoconstriction: a decrease in blood vessel diameter, usually caused by cryotherapy modalities.

Vasodilation: an increase in blood vessel diameter, usually caused by thermal modalities.

Venous stasis ulcer: an area of tissue breakdown that results from impaired venous return.

Vibration: massage technique in which the clinician provides a tremulous movement to cause the tissue to vibrate.

Viscosity: the thickness or resistance to flow of a fluid; the more viscous a fluid, the thicker it is.

Voltage: the force or pressure of electricity; produces an electrical force capable of moving charged particles through a conductor; noted as V and measured in volts (V).

W

Watt (W): a measure of power that is the rate at which work is done when 1 ampere (A, amp) of current flows through an electrical potential difference of 1 volt (V).

Waveforms: the visual representation of the variation of voltage over time.

Working pressure: pressure produced by active muscles pushing against an inelastic bandage.

REFERENCE

1.   Melzack R, Wall PD. Pain mechanisms: a new theory. *Science.* 1965;150(3699):971-979.

Key Abbreviations

A

ADL   activities of daily living
APTA   American Physical Therapy Association

B

BNR   beam nonuniformity ratio

C

CDC   Centers for Disease Control and Prevention
CHF   congestive heart failure
CVA   cerebrovascular accident

D

DOMS   delayed-onset muscle soreness
DVT   deep vein thrombosis

E

EMG   electromyographic biofeedback
ERA   effective radiating area

F

FES   functional electrical stimulation
FIR   far infrared

Memolo J.
Therapeutic Agents for the Physical Therapist Assistant
(pp 169-171). © 2022 SLACK Incorporated.

H

HVPC   high-voltage pulsed-current electrical stimulation

I

IASTM   instrument-assisted soft-tissue mobilization
IFC   interferential current therapy
IFR   infrared
IR   infrared

L

LED   light emitting diode
LLLT   low-level laser therapy

M

MIRE   monochromatic infrared energy
MS   multiple sclerosis

N

NIDA   National Institute on Drug Abuse
NMES   neuromuscular electrical stimulation

P

PAG   periaqueductal gray
PENS   patterned electrical neuromuscular stimulation
PICO(T)   patient, intervention, comparison, outcome, time
Pre-Mod   premodulated interferential current therapy
PSI   pounds per square inch
PSWD   pulsed shortwave diathermy

R

RCTs   randomized controlled trials
ROM   range of motion

S

SATA   spatial average temporal average intensity
SATP   spatial average temporal peak
SG   substantia gelatinosa
SWD   shortwave diathermy

T

TBI   traumatic brain injury
TENS   transcutaneous electrical nerve stimulation

U

UVA	ultraviolet A light
UVB	ultraviolet B light
UVC	ultraviolet C light

V

| VO_2 | maximal oxygen uptake |

W

| W/cm^2 | watts per centimeter squared |

Photo Credits

The figures below have been reproduced with permission from the respective manufacturer:

- **Accelerated Care Plus:** Figures 10-19, 10-20
- **DJO Global:** Figures 2-2, 2-5, 2-10, 2-11, 3-2, 4-7, 5-5, 5-11, 7-1, 7-2, 7-3, 7-4, 8-2, 8-14, 8-15, 10-8, 10-14, 10-21, 10-22, 10-23, 10-24, 10-25, 11-1, 11-2, 11-3, 11-4, 11-5, 11-6, 12-2, 12-3, 12-4
- **Lohmann & Rauscher:** Figure 8-3
- **Mettler Electronics Corporation:** Figure 10-15
- **OPTP:** Figure 6-4
- **Parker Laboratories:** Figure 5-12
- **Richmar:** Figures 5-6, 5-7, 10-9, 10-10
- **Thought Technology Ltd:** Figures 2-9, 10-26, 10-27

Index

CPSIA information can be obtained
at www.ICGtesting.com
Printed in the USA
BVHW010330110722
641601BV00005B/8